YOU CAN
RELIEVE PAIN

YOU CAN RELIEVE PAIN

How Guided Imagery
Can Help You Reduce Pain or
Eliminate It Altogether

Ken Dachman
and John Lyons

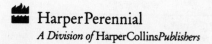

HarperPerennial
A Division of HarperCollins*Publishers*

A hardcover edition of this book was published in 1990 by
Harper & Row, Publishers.

First HarperPerennial edition published 1991.

Designer: Erich Hobbing
Illustrations by Ashamti Khan, One East Graphic Group, Inc.

The Library of Congress has catalogued the hardcover edition as
follows:

Dachman, Ken
   You can relieve pain : how guided imagery can help you
reduce pain or eliminate it altogether / Ken Dachman & John
Lyons.—1st ed.
      p. cm.
   Bibliography: p.
   ISBN 0-06-016054-3
      1. Intractable pain—Treatment.   2. Imagery (Psychology).
3. Intractable pain—Psychosomatic aspects.   I. Lyons, John
(John S.)   II. Title.
RB127.D33   1990
616'.0472—dc20   89-45032

ISBN 0-06-092023-8 (pbk.)
91 92 93 94 95 FG 10 9 8 7 6 5 4 3 2 1

K.D.

In loving memory of Rose Schuffler Dachman. Just being with her took my hurts away.

J.L.

To Cyndi, Trevor, and Caitlin with love.

Contents

List of Illustrations   *viii*

Acknowledgments   *ix*

1. The Eye of the Storm   1

2. Putting Pain into Focus   7

3. Blinded by the Pain   17

4. Controlling the Mind's Eye   25

5. A New Vision   39

6. A Sharper Image   55

7. Zeroing In: Pain-Control Imagery   87

8. Focusing on Relaxation   105

9. A Clear View: Using Your New Control   115

10. Other Vantage Points   125

Appendix: Support Groups and
          Other Organizations   145

Suggested Reading   153

Index   157

List of Illustrations

Pain-Control Scale   3

Mind-Body Communication   33

Central Nervous System   35

An "Involuntary" Action (Autonomic
    Nervous System)   37

A Safe Haven   120

Acknowledgments

Many thanks to John Whalen, Vince Tornatore, and Wayne Swanson for their highly skilled assistance in putting all this together.

And to Dr. Mark McGovern of Northwestern University for letting me apprentice under his skillful and patient tutelage.

Also to Dr. M. Willson Williams of the Union Institute. Her warm words of encouragement made a great and lasting impact.

And my deepest appreciation to Ed Hershman of Illinois Home Health Services, whose professionalism should serve as a model of conduct for all health care providers. Ed's humanity is well known to those fortunate enough to be in his life, and his friendship and generosity have inspired me.

KEN DACHMAN

YOU CAN
RELIEVE PAIN

CHAPTER 1

The Eye of the Storm

Pleasure is oft a visitant; but pain clings cruelly to us.

—JOHN KEATS

"My pain is like a powerful, relentless hurricane that rages wildly, battering my very foundation."

These are the exact words one of our patients used to describe the chronic pain that had devastated her life for thirteen years. They are also an appropriate metaphor for the process you are about to begin.

As anyone who has been trapped near a hurricane can attest, it is a terrifying, merciless, unpredictable juggernaut—a monster hundreds of miles wide, thousands of feet high, capable of inflicting unbelievable havoc and desolation.

The monster blasts ashore, shredding everything in its path—crushing buildings, snapping trees in half. The storm's victims huddle in shelters and basements, helpless against the assault of an awesome power that is beyond their understanding.

For too many who suffer with chronic pain, forces not unlike hurricane winds make life a daily battle against seemingly overwhelming odds. Our fragile armor of skin and bone is, after all, meager protection against a hurricane.

Ironically, at the center of a hurricane's murderous spiral—in the eye of the storm—all is calm. Winds are light and pleasant; the air is clean and dry. Often, the sun is shining.

This book will guide you to the serene center of the storms of pain that rage inside your body. Deep within you is a tranquil sanctuary. From this unique vantage point you'll be able to rally the skill and energy necessary to control and, perhaps, banish chronic pain from your life.

The journey to the eye of the storm will be an arduous passage, one that you must make alone. But we can guide you and help you gather the strength you'll need to reach your destination.

The process you'll learn is not grounded in religious faith, exotic mysticism, or parapsychological sorcery. No extraordinary talent is required—just a measure of hope and a willingness to try something new. The skills you'll develop as you work your way through this book will help you focus and refine a natural mechanism we all possess: the ability to control our lives by using our minds.

We wish we could grab your hand and lead you

where you need to go. We can't. It's not that easy. But you can reach the eye of the storm, and you will. We'll go slowly, moving carefully through four vital phases—understanding, training, practice, and execution.

The Pain-Control Scale offers a glimpse of what lies ahead. What if this device were all you needed to reduce your pain?

Sounds too easy, doesn't it? Yet a pain-control scale—or another image you conjure up in your own mind—may be the key to relieving your chronic pain,

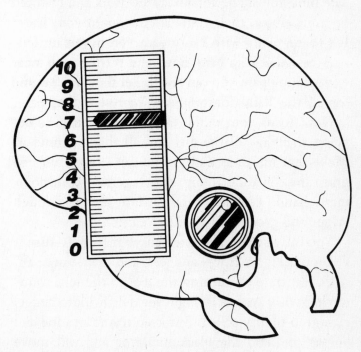

Pain-Control Scale

if you will let it. Take a few minutes now to learn to operate the scale. You'll want to return to it in the days and weeks ahead to measure the growing effectiveness of your pain-control abilities.

Imagine that the scale is your control panel, linked to an extremely sophisticated computer data bank—your brain. Stored in the data bank are intricately detailed sensory impressions of every pain you have ever experienced. The time you fell off your bicycle and broke your arm? It's there. The time you slammed the front door on your finger? It's there. The time you slipped on an icy sidewalk and bounced on your elbow, then your tailbone, then your back? It's there, along with every pain you have ever felt.

Access that data bank now, and retrieve the most excruciating pain you can recall. Let the no. 10 at the top of the Pain-Control Scale represent that pain.

Now, focus your mind. Use all your senses to develop an image of the dial and all that's behind it. Make that image as real as you can. Reach out and grasp the control dial with the fingers of your dominant hand. Feel its metal surface and the rough ridges and grooves of its outer edges.

You can use the dial to lessen your pain, to turn it down until it hurts less and less, and then, not at all.

Concentrate on turning the dial to the left, counterclockwise. At first it might seem difficult to budge, rigid, too tightly coiled. But keep trying. As the dial begins to turn, the black indicator bar will move slowly downward . . . millimeter by millimeter. Yes, it's slow going, but be patient. You'll hear a faint "click" as you move to each new level on the scale, accompanied by a perceptible decrease in the magnitude of your pain.

Don't worry if you're not able to move the indicator much. Most people find limited success in their first attempt. The first time you tried to walk you probably ended up face down in the rug, but that failure didn't stop you, did it? You tried again, and again, until you got it right.

You trained yourself to walk, and you can train yourself to control your chronic pain. It's possible to turn down your pain as easily as you turn down the volume on your car radio. It's possible to make this control as natural as walking, and as automatic as your millionth step.

Let's get started—after a note of caution: the skills you'll acquire through this book are intended to complement, not replace, your medical treatment.

CHAPTER 2

Putting Pain into Focus

> *All that is comes from the mind, it is based on the mind, it is fashioned by the mind.*
> —from the *Dhammapada* in the Pali Canon, the sacred scripture of Theravada Buddhism

The National Institute of Health estimates that chronic pain afflicts at least 90 million Americans, and counts among its victims those who suffer migraine headaches, back pain, arthritis, trauma, and catastrophic illness.

Pain is the primary reason for most visits to the doctor. Its treatment costs our economy close to $90 billion annually in medical expenses and lost productivity. (It is said that a nickel from the sale of each U.S. postage stamp is used to pay for postal workers' back pain!)

But what is pain?

You're looking for that goofy gravy boat that you got as a wedding present—the one you never use except when the friend who gave it to you comes to dinner. It's on the top shelf of the least accessible cabinet in your kitchen. You're not eight feet tall, so you can't reach it. You grab a chair and climb up on the counter. You reach for the gravy boat, accidentally dislodging an avalanche of Vego-Matics and super juicers and lazy susans. The rarely used kitchen paraphernalia surprises you. You lose your balance. You fall.

Suddenly you've entered the world of chronic pain.

Off you go to the doctor, and the doctor asks, "So where does it hurt?"

Is it that simple? Is pain simply where it hurts? Sometimes.

Acute pain, the sensation that accompanies injury, is a natural function, a warning that something is wrong with the body. Pain keeps us from showering under scalding water or ignoring a burst appendix or shattering a sprained ankle by walking on it. Pain alerts us to seek treatment for a fracture, a diseased gallbladder, a concussion.

Whenever your body is threatened by disease or hard contact with the sharp corners of the world, you experience acute pain.

Chronic pain (also known as intractable pain) doesn't serve the same purpose as acute pain. Chronic pain tells us that something's wrong, but it doesn't necessarily focus on any particular injury or part of the body. A migraine, for instance, rarely means that there's something wrong with the brain. Chronic pain is a signal, but of what? The truth is, no one knows, and that renders conventional medical treatments generally ineffective.

If you suffer from chronic pain you have probably visited a squadron of doctors, swallowed a pharmacy shelf full of drugs, and considered (or undergone) surgery. And still the pain persists. Angina. Dystrophy. Arthritis. Gout. Bursitis. Reynaud's disease. Fibrositis. Migraines. Shingles. Ulcers. Tendonitis. Lumbar pain. Neuralgia. Systemic pain. Tennis elbow. Housemaid's knee. Neuroma. Colitis. Myofibrositis. An oppressive, seemingly endless litany of suffering.

The U.S. Department of Health and Human Services has identified several major categories of chronic pain: arthritic, cancer, lower back, headache, neurogenic (damaged nerves), and psychogenic (pain with no apparent physical cause). Dr. John Loeser of the International Association for the Study of Pain simplifies the classification process greatly, dividing chronic pain into that which can be attributed to physical causes and that which can't.

The millions who suffer the ravages of chronic pain realize that having their symptoms diagnosed and categorized brings little comfort. Even so, it is beneficial for every chronic pain sufferer to learn all he or she can about the pain. As we'll see later, this knowledge can become an essential element in an effective control strategy.

It is extremely important that the government's primary health agency has created an official designation for pain with no discernible physical cause. What is now labeled "psychogenic pain" used to be called "psychosomatic pain." This class of pain, because it couldn't be isolated through X ray or CAT scan or other diagnostic hardware, was frequently blamed on the patient. "You're bringing this all on yourself," doctors would scold. "It's all in your head."

Psychogenic pain was thought to be unreal, evidence of extreme hypochondria, a pathetic plea for attention, a malingerer's malady, or a sign of mental disorder. Fortunately, medical science has become much more sophisticated over the past two decades, and a lot more humble. It now almost universally recognizes that pain is pain. If you hurt, you hurt, regardless of what tests, films, or sonar can find.

Further, it has become clear that so-called psychogenic pain usually has very real physical manifestations. We recently treated a patient suffering from irritable bowel syndrome (nervous stomach). This patient isn't at all adept in coping with stress of any kind. Like a bridge overloaded with traffic, her nerves snap under the weight of living. She grew up hesitant and anxious and has matured into an extremely skittish, severely depressed woman. Whenever one of her many fears and anxieties overwhelms her, this woman experiences severe pain in her abdomen. We have seen her stomach swell to several times its normal size during one of these attacks, as if she had become six months pregnant in a matter of minutes—a sad but dramatic illustration of the mind's effect on the body's interpretation of pain.

The fact that psychogenic pain clearly exists offers a bright ray of hope for all chronic pain sufferers. If our minds can make us sick, clearly a mind-body connection is at work. Can't that same connective tissue be used to make us well? Yes, it can. We can learn to exploit the interdependence of mind and body to control chronic pain—no matter what its source.

We need to learn pain control because medical science finds chronic pain difficult to treat effectively. Surgery, electrical stimulation, nerve blocks, and an arsenal of drugs have been tried, with little or no success.

Pain has become a multibillion-dollar industry. People will try just about anything in the hope of finally ridding themselves of pain. But all the new drugs that are discovered, all the new medical procedures that are perfected, and all the new technological devices that are invented may not improve on the one device readily available to all pain sufferers—the mind.

You have probably tried one form, if not several forms, of treatment to rid yourself of your pain. Each has its validity, and we encourage you to take advantage of all that medical science and technology makes available to you. However, we also encourage you to take advantage of your mind, the most advanced medical tool ever conceived. You can use it in combination with other therapies, and you can use it to do many of the same things the other treatments do, without some of their risks and side effects.

For example, drugs provide a necessary respite from agony for many chronic pain sufferers. Sadly, however, many pain-control drugs trigger side effects much more dangerous than the discomfort they are intended to treat. About 30 percent of prescription-drug users experience negative reactions to their medications. These reactions range from nausea and dizziness to hallucinations and addiction. An estimated 160,000 Americans die each year because of adverse reactions to a drug or a combination of drugs. Doctors have now become so concerned over drug-related malpractice claims that they provide each patient with a long list of possible side effects. Often enough to be troublesome, these lists can become self-fulfilling prophecies, and thousands of patients develop precisely the symptoms they've been warned against.

Over time, many pain patients develop a dependence on pain-killing drugs and on the various sleep aids often prescribed in tandem. We don't find this particularly surprising. A current television commercial presents a young lady kissing her Excedrin bottle. She loves her little pain reliever; how could she live without it? We get the impression that she couldn't. The bottle should be attached to a gold charm she can wear around her neck—an amulet to ward off all evil.

Painkillers prescribed on an "as needed" ("prn," from the Latin "pro re nata") basis encourage this kind of blatant overreliance on pharmaceuticals. Soon a patient finds himself or herself administering preventive doses—using prescription drugs to treat the fear of pain rather than the pain itself.

Long-term dependency on drugs eventually builds blood-chemistry tolerance to the medication's therapeutic qualities. Larger and more dangerous doses are required for less and less relief. The patient is ultimately left with the pain—and a drug habit. There's also strong evidence to indicate that extended drug usage seriously erodes the efficiency of the body's natural pain-suppression mechanisms. Clearly, as valuable as drugs have proven to be in the treatment of thousands of diseases, they offer no long-term solution to the problem of chronic pain.

What if you could use your mind as a drug? The fact is, you can. And the mind's therapeutic qualities can be administered as and when you like, free of charge and without uncomfortable side effects.

Another common pain treatment is nerve blocks. Nerve blocks are an attempt to treat chronic pain by interrupting the body's pain transmission network. The novocaine injection you receive at the dentist's office is a nerve block—a local anesthetic that temporarily prevents pain impulses from reaching the brain. Chronic pain patients who have undergone nerve blocks report varying degrees of relief. For some, pain subsides for only a few hours. Others, primarily patients with musculoskeletal problems, find that repeated nerve blocks sometimes produce progressively longer periods of relief. For most chronic pain patients, unfortunately, nerve blocks offer no permanent—or even long-term—relief.

Your mind is a most effective nerve block because it allows you to consciously redirect nerve impulses.

Surgery is often a viable treatment for pain. Obviously operations that target a specific cause of pain (removal of a diseased appendix, replacement of an arthritic joint, and the like) are now routine and usually effective.

However, neurological procedures, which involve the cutting or removal of nerves that transmit pain to the brain, can induce a number of nasty complications. Postoperative problems can include paralysis, palsy, and, more typically, numbness, which has sometimes proven to be more uncomfortable than the pain it replaces. Worse, for many patients, the original pain frequently returns within a year. The risks and limited effectiveness of neurological surgery make these procedures treatments of last resort.

An alternative to neurosurgery is electrical stimulation, which offers three slightly different approaches to pain control. One procedure involves surgical implantation of tiny electrodes in the pain-

inhibiting areas of the brain. These electro
then connected to a portable activation device ou
the body. Whenever pain reaches an unbeara
level, electrical stimulation is employed to block the
sensation in the brain. Although this procedure has
provided significant relief in many cases, it hasn't
been 100 percent effective, nor have its benefits been
lasting. The radical implantation technique carries all
the risks and potential postoperative problems of any
neurosurgery.

A second device is the Dorsal Column Stimulator
(DCS), which consists of electrodes and a radio re-
ceiver surgically implanted in the dorsal column areas of the spinal cord. When intense pain occurs, the
patient triggers a small antenna connected to a
battery-powered transmitter. A signal is received by
the DCS, and pain is relieved. No one knows why.
The device has limited value for only a small group of
chronic pain patients. It appears to be another treatment in which the dangers of major surgery usually
outweigh the likelihood of permanent pain relief.

A third electrical stimulation device became popu-
lar in the early 1970s—the Transcutaneous Nerve
Stimulator (TNS). A typical TNS mechanism includes small electrodes taped directly to the skin in
the painful area and a portable stimulator that pro-
duces an electronic pulse specially calibrated to reduce the patient's specific pain. Moderate to total
relief has been experienced by TNS users. The device
seems most effective in the treatment of neck, shoul-

der, and back pain. Unfortunately, long-term relief is not assured. Some TNS patients develop a tolerance of the device's stimulation; others find TNS to be of no help at all.

These techniques use technology to shock pain into submission. We contend you can use your mind to do it yourself.

Isn't it strange that we look to pharmacists, surgeons, technicians, and technology for answers that may be staring us in the face every time we look in the mirror?

The most effective treatment for chronic pain can't be found in a bottle or in a hospital operating room or at Radio Shack.

It lies within ourselves.

CHAPTER 3

Blinded by the Pain

PATIENT: Doc, it hurts when I do this.
DOCTOR: Then, don't do that.
                   —A classic vaudeville joke

It is so difficult for many chronic pain sufferers to exercise control over their pain—or even to *believe* that they can gain control—because pain has such a tremendous influence on their lives. Most spend from 80 to 90 percent of their waking hours thinking about their pain, or, more specifically, the impact pain is having on their lives—how it makes them feel, how it affects their relationships with family and friends, how it constricts and limits their activities, how much money it is costing them.

One of our patients provides a startling example of the impact of pain.

Charlotte is overweight and suffering from severe lower back pain.

Charlotte's first serious lumbar spasm occurred almost ten years ago. She was terrified. Her fears changed her life completely, overwhelming every aspect of her existence. She bought a hospital bed and installed it in her living room, close to the front door, to provide easy access to the ambulances she expected to come frequently.

Over time, Charlotte added traction pulleys to her bed, and then a sleeping board, and eventually an impressive collection of medical paraphernalia.

Next to her bed, Charlotte collected hundreds of pills: painkillers, tranquilizers, muscle relaxants, sleeping aids.

Charlotte may as well have been lying in a straitjacket as lying in a bed in her living room. She had tied herself up, exiled herself to her own house. She had created an environment that anticipated the impact of her back pain, and in the process she taught her mind a fantasy of pain that allowed her back spasms to dominate her life.

Admittedly, Charlotte is an extreme case. Even so, her withdrawal from life offers a valid warning—if you let chronic pain consume your life, it will.

For too many pain sufferers, the list of things that it hurts to do expands daily until it includes most of the activities in their lives. Brick by brick, the prison walls rise.

Fortunately, the same mental apparatus that allows some of us to embrace pain as a way of life can be used to rally the inner resources we need to gain control of pain and take back our lives.

An important aspect of learning to control your pain is an understanding of the true impact of pain on your daily life. To what extent does pain interfere with living? The Pain Behavior Assessment provides an accurate gauge of behaviors and feelings that can be attributed to the chronic pain experience.

The self-assessment has two purposes. First, it allows you to see, graphically, how much of your life you've given up to pain. Second, it allows you to monitor the progress you make with the pain-control program presented in this book.

Complete the assessment now, and again in six months. Your scores will provide you with an objective measure of your success, a way to compare your life now and after you've taken control of your pain. We believe you'll see a marked difference.

PAIN BEHAVIOR ASSESSMENT

Answer the following questions in terms of how you have felt about pain during the past month. Circle "yes" or "no" on this page or write down your answers on a separate sheet of paper:

YES no 1. I change my body position frequently.

YES no 2. I can stand for only a short period of time.

YES no 3. I go out less than I did previously.

YES   no   4. I sleep or nap more during the day.

YES   no   5. I spend a good deal of the day lying down to rest.

YES   no   6. I often say how bad or useless I am, or that I am a burden.

YES   no   7. I often moan, groan, or sigh from my pain or discomfort.

YES   no   8. I keep rubbing or holding areas of my body that hurt.

YES   no   9. I am irritable and impatient with myself.

YES   no   10. I require help to get into cars, bathtubs, and so on.

YES   no   11. I feel that I am always in a restricted position.

YES   no   12. I have trouble dressing myself (for instance, shoes, socks).

YES   no   13. I move slowly and carefully all the time.

YES   no   14. When I work, I do so in short bursts and then rest.

YES   no   15. I am doing less around the house than I used to.

YES   no   16. I am not using public transportation.

YES   no   17. I stay home much of the time.

YES   no   18. I am less interested in listening to other people's problems.

YES   no   19. I don't visit others as often as I used to.

YES   no   20. I am often irritable with people around me.

YES   no   21. My sexual activity has decreased.

YES   no   22. I am not doing the things I usually do to take care of my children or family.

YES   no   23. I walk shorter distances and stop more often to rest.

YES   no   24. I am more demanding of others than I used to be.

Today's Date ___ / ___ / ___   Score _____

Here's how to score this test. For each question answered with a "yes," give yourself one (1) point. Total your points and write your score in the space provided.

Remember to repeat the assessment in six months and compare your scores.

The following table indicates the extent to which chronic pain is affecting the quality of your life.

Score	Interference
20 or more	extreme
11 to 19	severe
6 to 10	moderate
3 to 5	mild
0 to 2	no interference

If you scored 2 points or less, congratulations. You've been able to keep pain from having a significant impact on your life. In our research, less than 5 percent of chronic pain sufferers reported life interference at this level.

If, like most respondents, you scored 3 or more points, you can begin to see what a destructive force chronic pain is. The problem, obviously, is not simply the sensation of pain, the hurt. The problem is the effect of pain on all the things you do or want to do every day. About 93 percent of pain sufferers score in the 3- to 19-point range.

Remember to write your score in the space provided. At this point, that number is a baseline, a starting point. By comparing this score to your score after you've mastered the pain-control protocol, you'll be able to determine exactly how much the technique has helped to make pain less central in your life.

TAKING CHARGE

Before you can begin to take control of your chronic pain, you must examine your perceptions of the pain experience.

First, realize that your pain is not some externally generated force sent to torment you by an enemy, or divine whimsy, or rotten luck. It's certainly not a punishment for past sins. And it's not a foreign object that slipped inside you one night as you slept. Your pain is part of you, a message from your innermost self.

You must take responsibility for your pain; you must admit ownership. Your pain is yours. It's important to know this, to admit it. Knowing that your pain is uniquely yours will help you to manage it. Don't confuse responsibility with blame. If you blame yourself for your pain, it's easy to see the pain as penance, something you deserve, an agony you must endure. If you blame your pain on some external force, you could fall into a victim mentality, seeing yourself abused and tortured by some force beyond your control. You'll see no hope for change—or even escape—and spend precious energy and time on self-pity. You'll accept your suffering, using it as an excuse to withdraw, to give up. For some, there's self-destructive comfort in being a victim. A victim doesn't have to do anything—except suffer.

Acceptance of a victim's role is not always the fault of the pain sufferer. Many who suffer from chronic pain find themselves caught up in a tragic phenomenon: victim bashing. Your family and friends become annoyed, or frustrated, or simply angry with the behavioral effects of your chronic pain. They begin blaming you for failing to deal with your pain properly. "It can't possibly be that bad," family and friends believe (because they're not experiencing the pain). There are even therapists who participate in victim bashing, beginning treatment with questions like "why did you choose your pain?" It's not difficult to understand why many pain sufferers eventually join in the victim bashing themselves, blaming themselves for their pain and convincing themselves that they are doomed. Depression, despair, and bitterness follow, overwhelming the desire to try and recapture control of their lives.

Equally destructive is the stoic, almost saintly posture adopted by some pain sufferers. Trained (conditioned is a better word) from childhood to accept life without complaint, these noble souls grin—or grimace—and bear their pain like a badge of honor. These people make no attempt to manage their pain. Their doctors advise these remarkable folks to live with the pain, so they do—miserably.

These counterproductive attitudes must be banished or no pain-control program can have any chance of success.

The first step is to take responsibility for your pain. Recognize its causes without assigning blame. Assume full ownership. Although you don't want your pain, admit it's yours. Once you accept ownership, the concept of control is easy to grasp. If your pain is yours, a part of you, you can control it, just as you control other aspects of your self—your physical movements, your speech, your behavior, and so on. You don't need to rely on high-tech apparatus or other people to fix what's uniquely yours.

For some people, admitting ownership of pain is a scary proposition. Their victim's or saint's cloak feels comfortable. It's easy to blame chronic pain for all their troubles in life. If you are responsible for yourself and make the commitment to participate in your own treatment, you are leaving the sidelines and entering the game. And if you don't play, you can't win.

CHAPTER 4

Controlling the Mind's Eye

> *So great a power is there of the soul upon the body, that whichever way the soul imagines and dreams that it goes, thither doth it lead the body.*
>
> —AGRIPPA

All experience, including the experience of pain, is in the domain of the mind. This was clear two thousand years ago to the Roman general and statesman Marcus Vipsanius Agrippa, and it has been understood perfectly in several Eastern cultures for even longer. The message is validated daily by modern pain-control experts across the United States and around the world.

In simple language, all pain is subjective. It's a personal perception. What hurts one person may not bother you a bit. And the pain that wracks you today might seem to disappear tomorrow. Pain is whatever the mind decides it is.

In Western cultures, there are numerous examples of the mind's power to control pain. During World War II, for instance, Dr. H. K. Beecher treated the battle wounds of U.S. soldiers. He discovered that only a third of the seriously wounded soldiers experienced enough pain to request morphine. Then, after the war, Beecher treated civilian patients who had wounds as severe as those suffered by the soldiers. Yet nearly 80 percent of these patients needed morphine to control their pain. Why? Beecher, in his widely quoted research, found that the soldiers responded to their wounds with "relief, thankfulness at the escape alive from the battlefield, even euphoria," rather than pain. He theorized that the civilians saw their wounds as "depressing, calamitous" events.

G. Gordon Liddy, the famous Watergate conspirator, described in his book *Will* how he would hold his hand directly over an open flame to demonstrate his inner strength. The trick, Liddy claimed, was "not to mind" the pain. We suspect that Liddy "minded" his pain quite a bit, enough to control the effects the heat from the flame should have had on his body.

Liddy's demonstration seems trivial when compared with the pain-control exploits of Jack Schwarz. Burning cigarettes pressed into Schwarz's flesh elicit no cries of pain and produce no blisters. Pain researchers have pushed five-inch-long needles through his arms. When the needles are extracted, no blood flows and no puncture marks are visible. Schwarz, who was a prisoner of the Nazis during World War II, discovered and developed his abilities to survive that horror.

Doctors Elmer and Alice Green of the Menninger Clinic in Topeka, Kansas, verified Schwarz's remarkable capabilities through extensive tests a decade ago. They have also examined many other talented controllers of the mind-body link. Research subjects have shown the ability to alter their heartbeats, direct blood circulation, block pain, control bleeding, raise and lower temperature, and dramatically accelerate the healing process. One of the Greens' subjects was able to create a small growth on his hand, *on request*. He could also cause the growth to dissolve.

While we tend to assign mystical or spiritual powers to those who can control their bodies through the mind, a majority of the most talented "controllers" studied during the past decades have been normal, otherwise unremarkable folks.

In 1965, a middle-aged Bulgarian underwent major surgery to repair a large hernia, *without anesthetic*. The patient remained conscious throughout the procedure and reported no pain. Bleeding was minimal during surgery and the man healed much faster than usual. We know this remarkable feat is credible because the operation was filmed and has since been studied at hundreds of medical schools. There was nothing unusual about the patient, an anonymous semiskilled laborer, except for the pain control he exhibited.

Vernon Craig, an Ohio cheesemaker, would tell observers "I'm just an ordinary man." Then he would walk barefoot over glowing hot coals, or make himself the filling in a nail-bed sandwich, or climb ladders whose rungs were razor-sharp sabers. At the conclusion of these amazing performances, no cuts, bruises, or blood ever appeared. Craig, as a child, had come across a yoga textbook. The author claimed that the mind could be trained to control pain. Craig proved that it could. When he strolled for twenty-five yards across coals burning at 1,494° Fahrenheit, this "ordinary man" earned a place in the *Guinness Book of World Records*.

Sports history is rich in stories of athletes who have overcome pain and injury to continue performing, often extremely well. Chicago Bears' quarterback Jim McMahon has played in severe pain for several years and has excelled. One of McMahon's predecessors, Bobby Douglas, once threw a seventy-yard touchdown pass with a broken arm. Mickey Mantle played baseball for more than a decade on legs mangled by injuries and outfield fences. Former heavyweight champion Muhammad Ali fought Ken Norton furiously, toe-to-toe, for seven rounds after Ali's jaw was broken.

Our morning newspapers offer more examples of the power of the mind. A victim of attempted murder runs more than a mile with three bullets in his back.

A father endures searing flames to rescue his daughter from a burning house. Tibetan monks hike miles through subzero mountain air clad only in loincloths.

The evidence is clear: the mind's extraordinary power can heal and soothe the body. Thousands of pain patients across the United States demonstrate these powers daily as they employ a variety of mind-based techniques to alleviate, manage, or subdue their chronic pain.

THE MIRACLE WITHIN

Dramatic testimony about the mind's power can be found in a recent psychological study of patients suffering multiple personality disorder. Researchers Dr. Frank W. Putnam, Juliet J. Guroff, Dr. Edward K. Silberman, Lisa Barban, and Dr. Robert M. Post studied 100 patients and found that, within the same person, alternate personalities frequently had differing pain symptoms, such as headaches, and had differing reactions to the same medications. Remarkably, some even had differing allergies.

Research has also proven that a long list of healing processes have been facilitated by "mind modulation" of various body tissues and cells. In *The Psychology of Healing*, E. L. Rossi gives an extensive summary that includes the following:

- headache relief
- blood coagulation in hemophiliacs

- amelioration of hypertension
- amelioration of cardiac problems
- enhancement of the immune response
- healing of burns and bruises
- control of bleeding during surgery
- improvement of Reynaud's disease

Mind modulation has even been reported to cure warts. It's important to emphasize that Rossi's list is not a "Ripley's Believe It or Not" collection of isolated oddities. Most of the mind-aided healings Rossi cites have been duplicated successfully in strictly controlled laboratory settings.

Rossi and several other psychobiologists assert that mind-based therapies are effective because they influence the hypothalamus, a tiny region of the brain that regulates most of our allegedly "involuntary" maintenance functions (heartbeat, breathing, circulation, blood pressure, etc.). Nerve fibers from almost all other areas of the brain enter the hypothalamus, so there is a physical network capable of carrying mind-body communications. These messages trigger the stimulation of blood flow, the increase or decrease in gastrointestinal activity, or the regulation of body temperature. Lending credence to the theory is the recent discovery of a direct connection between the hypothalamus and immune system via limbic-hypothalamic pathways (Rossi, 1986). In laboratory studies with guinea pigs, lesions of the hypothalamus have been found to suppress certain immune functions.

"The mind," Ernest Rossi states in *Psychobiology of Mind-Body Healing*, "can regulate functions within the cells of all major organ systems and tissues of the body via the autonomic nervous system." He believes that the intricate interactions between mind and body, which extend down to the cellular level, may take us decades to completely understand. Yet Rossi is convinced that such interactions occur regularly in a three-stage process through which the mind activates and manages "hundreds of incredibly complex biochemical reactions."

In stage one of the regulatory process, the mind generates images in the cerebral cortex. In stage two, these images are filtered through the hypothalamus, in the form of neural impulses. They emerge as neurotransmitters, or "messenger molecules," capable of influencing functions of the autonomic nervous system. Stage three finds these messenger molecules such as serotonin and adrenaline triggering biochemical changes such as improved circulation and more efficient metabolism within individual body cells.

Evidence suggests that the success of pain control through this mental intervention process may involve the stimulation of the production of biochemical substances called *endorphins*. Researchers attempting to determine why morphine was such an effective analgesic accidentally discovered endorphins ("the morphine within") in 1975. These natural painkillers, ten times as potent as morphine, are manufactured by our bodies.

Two other endogenous substances—epinephrine, a stimulant, and norepinephrine, a relaxant—have frequently been detected in blood-chemistry analyses associated with laboratory studies of the mind-body interaction.

The mind-body interaction seen by psychobiologists can be compared to the operation of a computer. The mind, like a computer programmer, creates operating instructions. The mind's instructions are in the form of imagery, while the computer's instructions are in the form of the numbers and symbols of the computer program. In the mind, the hypothalamus converts imagery into neural impulses, just as the computer's central processing unit converts programs into electronic impulses. Finally, the body's organs, tissues, and cells understand and act upon the impulses they receive, just as the computer's operating circuits do.

The analogy is an extreme oversimplification of a complex multidimensional process we may never fully understand. Fortunately, we don't have to completely comprehend every intricate nuance of the mind-body communication process to take advantage of it. All we need to realize is that there is a structure which allows messages from the mind to reach and affect every cell of the body.

The key to mind-body communications is imagery. The sights, sounds, fragrances, tastes, and textures we experience through our physical senses are interpreted in the mind as images. These images define and regulate our existence and our relationship with our environment. Imagery provides the only "messages" our body's operating systems recognize and respond to. If we can control the imagery that constitutes our body's operating language, we can control pain.

To help you grasp the mind-body dynamics that you'll use to control your chronic pain, it is important to review some of the hundreds of complex

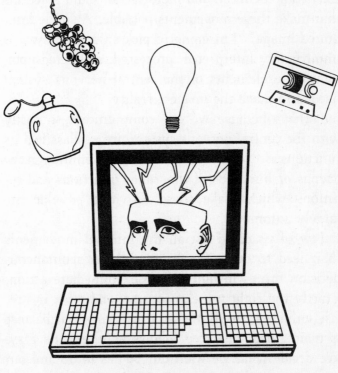

Mind-Body Communication

bodily functions you control every waking moment via the central nervous system. (The illustration on page 35 demonstrates one of the functions regulated through this infrastructure.) Most healthy humans are quite adept at controlling the functions activated through the central nervous system. It's a skill we've been practicing all our lives. We don't think about commanding our muscles to contract or relax when we stand up, sit down, wiggle our noses, or curl our toes. We certainly aren't intimidated by the complex electrical, chemical, and motor actions and reactions that make these movements possible. A single integrated image, "I'm going to pick an apple now," is immediately interpreted, processed, and acted upon by all the elements of the central nervous system needed to make the image a reality.

Perhaps because we can communicate so easily with the central nervous system, we've classified its functions as "voluntary" activities—even though the dozens or hundreds of thousands of actions and reactions which make these activities possible are largely automatic.

Few of us could list all the internal movements that need to occur for us to walk. A spontaneous decision brings instant response, immediate action. Exactly the right muscles contract and relax in precisely the best rhythm. Our arms swing, our balance is maintained, one step follows another. It's easy. We decide what we want our bodies to do and our bodies respond to our commands.

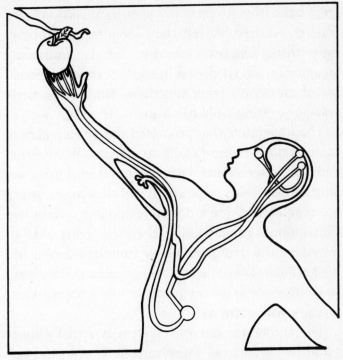

Central Nervous System

Why, then, can't we control *all* our physical functions as easily—including those related to the interpretation and transmission of pain?

We believe the answer can be found in our evolutionary history.

THE NEURODEVELOPMENTAL IMPERATIVE

When our prehistoric ancestors finally pulled themselves out of the primordial ooze, their needs were basic (though certainly pressing). Food. Water. Shelter. As they evolved, they developed control over only those functions required by the immediate struggle for survival—not because they were incapable of mastering other functions, but because there was no pressing need to do so.

The imperative that prompted the development of motor skills, hunting skills, and speech never prodded man to seek control over other internal processes such as heartbeat, respiration, and circulation, which are regulated by the autonomic nervous system (see illustration). Paradoxically, the intelligence that allowed man to dominate his environment diminished his need to manage his internal processes. Why learn to control our body temperature when animal skins and fire will warm us?

The autonomic nervous system is actually made up of two branches—the sympathetic and parasympathetic nervous systems. These two control many of the same organs but with very different effects.

In general, the sympathetic system activates a part of the body. For example, when a burst of energy is needed for a sudden activity, the heart beats faster, pupils dilate, and blood pumps harder.

The parasympathetic system usually restores calm to the body. Pupils contract, the heart slows down, and blood pressure normalizes. All this, apparently, without any conscious or voluntary intervention.

The theory of the neurodevelopmental imperative implies that the distinction between "voluntary" and

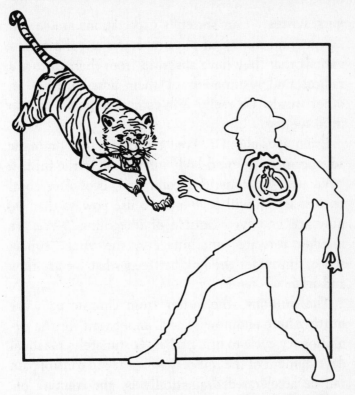

An "Involuntary" Action (Autonomic Nervous System)

"involuntary" functions is nothing more than a vestige of a distant evolutionary prioritization. The next step in our development could well include a neuro-imaginal imperative—the psychoneurological mediation of all internal functions through imagery.

We could be headed toward a universal mastery of capabilities we have always possessed. We are not alone in voicing this hope for the future. Dr. Robert Ornstein, author of *The Psychology of Conscious-*

ness, writes: "Our society's expectations are so low . . . mental control of physical states can show individuals that they have absorbed from their culture a radical underestimation of their possibilities." In other words, we really won't know what we can do until we try.

Brain specialist Dr. Frederic Tilney sees dramatic advancement in mind-body interaction in the future. "We will, by conscious command, evolve cerebral centers which will permit us to use powers that we now are not even capable of imagining." We are moving forward, and imagery, the vital "supersense," provides the link between what we are now and what we can be.

The millions who suffer from chronic pain are hurting here and now. They cannot wait for the evolutionary cycle to bring relief. Fortunately, personal development of the imagery necessary to control pain can be accelerated dramatically by the training offered later in this book. We will provide you with a concise formula for the effective use of guided imagery, a process with an impressive record of success.

CHAPTER 5

A New Vision

> *The mind of man is capable of any-*
> *thing—because everything is in it, all the*
> *past, as well as all the future.*
> —JOSEPH CONRAD

At the center of our being, in the "eye" of the soul, is a vibrant, vivid, incredibly powerful mechanism called imagery. Imagery is the source of an eclectic melange of sensory impressions and symbolic representations that define the way we truly "see" ourselves and the world.

We believe that imagery is our dominant sensory faculty and the mind's primary vehicle for interpreting, organizing, and processing experience. It employs the other senses, which we will refer to as *sensors*, as antennae to collect the raw data the mind uses to construct its world.

Imagery allows our sensors to operate as an integrated system of interpretation and response. The sights, sounds, tastes, smells, and textures our sensors accumulate are interpreted by the mind as imagery—the only language it understands.

Many of us think of imagery as strictly a visual process, but all the senses contribute to the mind's interpretation of experience. We contend that the imaginal process enables us to see ourselves as we really are, giving us a deeper, much more complete insight.

An image should not be thought of as just a mental photograph. Instead, it is a full-bodied, three-dimensional experience, complete with sounds, smells, tastes, and textures. For example, a Christmas snapshot of a family gathered around the tree is a pale shadow of the actual experience. Your mind's eye can create a much more richly detailed image. You can smell the crisp fragrance of the Scotch pine, taste the moist, flavorful turkey, hear the sweet voices of the children singing "Silent Night," and feel the warmth of a toddler's excited embrace.

In fact, visuals are not necessary for vivid imagery. One of the best imagers we encountered is a woman who has been blind since birth. Yet she understood imagery immediately. When she needed to relax, she quickly learned to let her mind take her to a warm, quiet beach where she could unwind. "I've never seen the ocean blue," she told us. "I don't know what blue looks like. But I've been on a boat, and breathed the sea air, and felt the spray. I know what blue feels like. And I know what the sand feels like, and the warmth of the sun." Obviously, therapists who refer to imagery as "movies of the mind" are severely constricting its depth and range.

An image can be seen, heard, smelled, felt, and tasted by the mind all at once. You can experience yourself from deep within your body or from a thousand miles up in space, or from both perspectives at once. You can be sitting at a table in your home and at the same time be climbing the Spanish steps in Rome, or crossing the Rockies in a hot-air balloon, and it takes no special creativity.

Because each of us is unique, so are our images. Your friend's image of "the best Christmas I ever experienced" is nothing like yours, despite the similar feelings each might inspire. Similarly, you might say to a friend, "Today's beautiful. The clouds are high and wispy, the sky's blue, it's warm. I feel great."

"Oh, I don't know," your friend replies. "I like cool, wet days better. I feel more romantic, mysterious. You feel the mist on your skin, you turn up your collar and walk into the fog like Bogart in *Casablanca*. That, to me, is a beautiful day."

The ability to create specific, focused images is something we all possess to some degree. It is a natural faculty that has been developed more effectively by some of us than others.

One of the most remarkable imagers of this century was Nikola Tesla. A creative scientific genius, he harnessed the electrical power of Niagara Falls and designed over 700 inventions including neon, fluorescent lighting, the oscillator, many of our basic electric motors, and several remote-control devices.

Tesla trained in imagery as a child, and he refined his faculties to the point where he was able to construct complicated inventions, in detail, *in his mind.* According to the machinists who actually constructed his inventions, Tesla could visualize each intricate detail in dimensions down to one ten-thousandth of an inch.

Author Thomas Wolfe attributed much of his writing ability to his highly developed sense of imagery. Describing an image of an iron railing along the boardwalk in Atlantic City, Wolfe wrote, "I could see it instantly, just the way it was, the heavy iron pipe; the raw galvanized look; the way the joints were fitted together. It was all so vivid and concrete that I could feel my hands upon it and know the exact dimensions, its size and weight and shape."

It is important, however, not to confuse imagery with imagination. Imagining, or fantasizing, is often aimless and unfocused. It is directed outside yourself and need not have any basis in reality. Imagery is much more focused. When you use pure imagery, you are using your primary sense. You can marshal the forces of your sensors to control the only thing in this world you can control: yourself—your own body and your own mind.

IMAGINAL LEARNING

It is ironic that imagery is not encouraged in our schools, except in creative writing and art classes. We believe that imagery is a fundamental element in the learning process. Experience and research have proven that the development of imagery improves memory and accelerates learning. In a number of pilot programs designed for children, for example, visual, auditory, and tactile aids to stimulate the imagination have increased learning skills from 20 to 30 percent.

Almost all early learning seems to require the use of imagery. How, for example, does a baby learn to walk? Does the baby read a manual, interview experienced walkers, follow verbal instructions from Mom and Dad? Not likely. A growing number of experts believe that our minds use imagery to teach our bodies to perform physical activities such as walking.

You crawled before you walked, and the data your sensors gathered as you crawled helped you gauge where you were in space and time. You felt the carpet beneath you. You groped your way along the edge of the table. You touched. You saw your parents or other people walk. You heard steps on the floor, which let you know the sounds your feet should make. All this sensing became for you the image of walking. Your sensors provided the input that your imaginal sense turned into a message for your mind. When your mind—and then your tiny body—began to understand the message, you tried your first step.

And fell down.

But your mind had created an image of what walking was supposed to be. You used this image to guide you as you tried again and again to walk, and eventually your physical movements matched the image. You walked. You were too young to be told, so you had to be shown. And you showed yourself. Imagery allowed you to understand where you wanted to go and how to get there.

Think about more complicated physical feats. Hitting a baseball traveling toward you at ninety miles an hour and likely to jump, drop, or curve at any moment requires an almost perfect integration of imagery and movement. Seasoned sluggers report "feeling" the ball to the bat.

The karate master's performance is a flashing ballet of kicks, spins, and jabs. Without an image to emulate, how does the master attain the incredible speed, precision, and beauty embodied in the art? How can he perform so instinctively, so spontaneously? Surely the mind choreographs each move the black belt makes.

Obviously, practice plays a role in perfecting physical skills. But as years of research have shown, imagery can advance and enhance the learning process.

In their excellent book, *Superlearning*, Sheila Ostrander and Lynn Schroeder describe an athletic training technique called *visualization*. This approach to preparation takes advantage of the fact that effective imagery can have as significant an impact as actual physical experience. In fact, it can be argued that imagery can even have a greater impact because there is no external interference to the imaging process. We don't particularly agree with the use of the term "visualization," however, since it emphasizes the visual aspect when in reality the technique employs all the sensors. Nevertheless, the technique itself has proven to be quite effective. It has been used successfully for decades in Soviet-bloc countries, and within the past few years it has become a part of U.S. Olympic training programs. Most sports scientists now believe that the average athlete will never realize even half of his or her potential unless some sort of mental training accompanies traditional practice.

To activate their visualizations (images), Eastern European athletes lie down and listen to soothing music. Within minutes, the athletes are deeply relaxed; their hearts beat in time to the music. The athletes then create in their minds a detailed image of a winning performance. They "see" (and hear and feel) themselves at their best. The hundreds of gold medals won in Olympic and world championship competitions by Soviet and East German athletes indicate how often the physical act duplicates the perfect image previously visualized. Research suggests that athletes who spend more of their time in mental training consistently perform better than those who emphasize purely physical preparation.

The millions who watched the 1988 Winter Olympics saw several downhill skiers using imagery to prepare for the biggest race of their lives. Standing on a wooden floor in the waiting area, these athletes used their minds to conquer the mountain waiting for them outside. Leaning, tucking, hurtling forward and easing back, the skiers anticipated each gate, each turn, each icy rise, each blast of powder. Imagery enabled the skiers to experience the course without ever leaving the room.

Professional golfer Jack Nicklaus claims that his success is *entirely* attributable to concentration and visualization. Body-builder-turned-movie-star Arnold Schwarzenegger maintains that, in weight lifting, the mind is everything. "As long as the mind can envision the fact that you can do something, you can," Schwarzenegger says. Dancers, acrobats, ice skaters, skiers, and basketball players all report similar satisfaction with imagery-assisted training. Imagery seems to be the language their bodies best understand.

IMAGERY AND "INVOLUNTARY" RESPONSE

We have harnessed the power of imagery to control so-called voluntary, physical functions instantaneously and naturally. Yet control of so-called involuntary or autonomic functions is a faculty underdeveloped in most of us, a capability that requires training and practice to perfect.

However, it can be done, as the experience of biofeedback therapists proves. The mind, through imagery, can regulate heartbeat, circulation, mobilization of the immune system, temperature, and several other functions traditionally labeled "involuntary" activities. A subject undergoing biofeedback training is linked to machinery that can measure internal activities through electrodes attached to various parts of the body. By invoking appropriate imagery, the subject is able to influence a wide range of biological functions. To reduce muscle tension, for example, the subject imagines floating in a quiet pool; to quicken heartbeat, he or she might run a mental marathon. The biofeedback machine's lights, bells, and displays instantly tell the subject how much control he or she is exerting. Originally, biofeedback technicians gave their hardware credit for the control exhibited by subjects. Yet biofeedback machinery no more induces the response than a stopwatch induces a world record time in the hundred-meter dash. It merely records the response. Research has proven that imagery activates the controlling impulses.

You have probably experienced imagery's effects on your internal physical functions hundreds or even thousands of times. Recall your most recent nightmare. Didn't your heartbeat accelerate? Didn't your breathing become quick and shallow? Wasn't that real adrenaline pumping through your body, and real perspiration dampening your chest? And weren't those very real physical responses activated by images—experiences that occurred only in your mind?

Think about what happens as you're nearing the end of a tough day. You've missed lunch, and you decide that you deserve a visit to your favorite restaurant.

You imagine the restaurant's specialty—a thick, lean, juicy New York strip steak, perfectly aged and elegantly prepared. And accompanying the steak is a plump, steaming baked potato, split in its center to form a warm, soft pocket for fresh butter and light sour cream. And there'll be a dish of your favorite vegetables, crispy green, laced with a hint of lemon, and a basket of the best golden-brown homemade bread you've ever had.

If you "see" that image clearly enough in your mind's eye, it will probably make your mouth water. Yet our salivary glands are considered to be involuntary mechanisms. You can tell yourself to salivate, but not much will happen. Instead, you have used imagery to stimulate salivation—a physical function not ordinarily under your control.

It's important to note that you aren't reacting to a *picture* of the meal; you are responding to your mind's uniquely comprehensive sensory image of the steak and its trimmings. The image includes a kaleidoscope of sensory data chosen and organized by your mind; the steak's appearance, aroma, and texture, the feeling of the knife in your hand as you cut into the tender meat, the sounds of the restaurant, the steam rising from the potato, the vivid colors of the vegetables. Your mind selected and organized elements of all these variables, and the resulting image sent your body a message it could not ignore.

Most of us are much too familiar with the impact of negative images on our bodies. We know from experience that it is indeed possible to "worry yourself sick." Consider the situation of the neophyte actor appearing on Broadway for the first time. It's opening night and he is extremely nervous. He finds himself imagining all the things that could go wrong. No one will laugh at his best jokes; they *will* laugh at his serious soliloquy. He'll forget his lines. He'll fall down, or his pants will. One hundred and forty terrible things will happen to him, he's sure of it. And as his mind sees the disasters ahead, the actor's stomach begins to churn. Soon, it becomes necessary for the actor to dash desperately to the bathroom—to deal with his body's physical reaction to the images his mind has created.

In our first example, a pleasant image triggered a pleasurable reaction in the body. In the second, an unpleasant mental prompt induced pain and discomfort. The point is clear: messages from our minds, if embedded in effective imagery, have a very real physical impact. Experts such as William Masters and Virginia Johnson have long maintained the importance of imagery in sexual performance, for example, which supports the axiom that the mind is indeed our greatest sexual organ.

You now know that imagery offers you access to the control of autonomic functions. But this knowledge takes you only a short distance down the path to the control of chronic pain. The imaging process must be refined and focused to take you the rest of the way.

IMAGERY IN PAIN CONTROL

The Western world's health care establishment has only recently acknowledged imagery as a valid and valuable technique for the management of chronic pain, even though imagery has been in use for centuries as a primary element in the disciplines of yoga, meditation, hypnosis, and psychotherapy.

Nevertheless, numerous Western doctors are now convinced that imagery is a powerful tool. Neurologist and neurosurgeon C. Norman Shealy, founder of the Pain Rehabilitation Center in La Crosse, Wisconsin, regards imagery as "the number one plan to stop pain. It is the single most effective technique, bar none." Dr. Neil Olshan, director of the Mesa (Arizona) Lutheran Hospital's Chronic Pain Control Unit, reports that 83 percent of patients who learned pain control imagery reduced their discomfort by 55 to 100 percent.

The specific tool these doctors are talking about is guided imagery—imagery specifically created and directed for therapeutic purposes. In our practice, we call it "clinical imagery" to draw attention to its role as a therapeutic tool in the treatment and control of pain and other symptoms. Numerous doctors have reported dramatic results when guided imagery has been used to treat a wide variety of medical problems, including cancer. Dr. Bernie Siegel, in his book *Love, Medicine, and Miracles*, describes the experience of a young patient afflicted with a brain tumor. The patient, a boy named Glen, learned imagery at the Mayo Clinic. At the suggestion of his therapists, Glen visualized a video game rocket ship blasting away at the tumor inside his head. After using this imagery for several weeks, Glen one day reported that he'd "gone on patrol" but could no longer find the tumor. A CAT scan couldn't find it either. It was gone, vaporized by Glen's imaginal rocket lasers, in combination with his other therapies.

Dr. David E. Bresler, director of the UCLA Pain Control Unit, has used guided imagery therapy extensively and reports: "In my experience, guided imagery has proven to be a safe and effective means of reprogramming the nervous system to maximize self-healing. Images are the language of the unconscious mind, and, when properly programmed, they are able to mobilize, to a remarkable degree, the body's intrinsic ability to heal itself."

One of Bresler's patients "saw" her facial pain as a

fire in her mouth. When Bresler asked her to think of ways to extinguish the fire, the woman created an image of cool clouds of water absorbing the flames, and her pain gradually subsided.

Dr. Nicholas Hall, of the George Washington Medical Center in Washington, D.C., found that imagery could be used by patients to significantly increase the number of circulating white cells and raise levels of several other internal substances known to increase the efficiency of the body's immune system. Similarly, Doctors Carl Simonton and Stephanie Mathews-Simonton of the Cancer Counseling Center in Fort Worth, Texas, have used guided imagery techniques in which cancer patients create images of white cells attacking diseased cells. This imaging process has reduced pain dramatically for many patients, shrunk tumors in others, and significantly extended the lives of several more.

In yet another application, a patient of Doctors Elmer and Alice Green at the Menninger Clinic in Topeka, Kansas, used imagery to treat the severe pain of pelvic cancer. The doctors asked the patient to create an image of "a room in his brain" that housed valves that controlled his blood supply. The patient "saw" the room and then found, and turned off, the valve that supplied blood to the tumor in his pelvis. The cancer eventually shrank to one-fourth its former size.

These and countless additional cases have proven that imagery is a powerful therapeutic tool. The examples also give you an idea of the wide range of ways imagery can be applied. The applications are nearly limitless, because the ways imagery affects our lives are nearly limitless. Imagery programs our dreams, enhances our fantasies, sharpens our recollections, and shapes our lives. Images can show us what we are and what we can be. By refining, focusing, and guiding your unique imaginal forces, you will be able to conquer your chronic pain.

CHAPTER 6

A Sharper Image

We can all image, and we all do, every day. Think about how you wince when you hear a car's brakes screech. Think about what a sponge feels like or what a cup of vinegar smells like. Your mind recognizes these images and responds to them—whether or not the car, the sponge, or the vinegar are really present.

All of us vary in our ability to use imagery skills, however. Some of us are All-Stars, and some of us belong on the sandlots. But if we work at it, we all have the chance to make it to the big leagues.

The most talented imagers are capable of focusing so strongly on an image that physical changes occur in their bodies. If a hypnotist, for example, suggests to one of these talented few that a pencil is a hot poker, skin blisters will appear where the pencil touches skin. Without training, the rest of us possess only fair imagery talents. Our minds image constantly to allow us to understand the world, but focused or guided imagery is a more difficult and more completely developed use of this imaging. In this chapter we will help you brush up on your imaging skills. First we will show you exercises that will help you rediscover just how powerful your sensors are. Then we will show you exercises to build your imaging talents so that you will be able to apply them to control your pain.

Why can some people focus their imaging better than others? Are they blessed? Have they made a deal with the devil? No. It's more likely that the great majority of us have simply been neglecting imagery, living too doggedly here and now in a world that seems to reward the logical, the analytical, and the articulate. Our society ignores, or worse, discourages sensory development.

Let us chase you back into your childhood for a moment. As a child, your life was self-centered and introspective. You were so focused on yourself and what you felt that you were constantly aware of your images and their effect on your life.

As children, we spent every waking (and dreaming) moment touching, tasting, sniffing, listening, and watching. We explored every corner of our lives, and we used imagery to understand what we found.

But then we went to school, where, instead of being encouraged to cultivate, strengthen, and enjoy our richest inner sense, we were transformed into information processors. We became collectors instead of explorers, forced to memorize, store, and recall fact after fact; we were trained to focus on the concrete reality of the external world rather than on our internal thoughts and feelings.

As adults, our imagery skills have fallen dormant. Fortunately, our ability to image is still with us. It's always been there, and it's never going to go away. Consider an accident victim whose leg has been in a cast for several months. He or she is often shocked when the cast is removed. The leg has atrophied, withered, and shrunk to perhaps half its normal thickness. Muscles are weak and difficult to control, and the joints are stiff and sore. Only concentrated rehabilitation can restore the leg to its natural state of strength and flexibility.

The same is true of imagery. You need to rehabilitate your imaging skill and feel again how much there is around you to experience every day. The imagery exercises in this chapter will help you to reactivate your imaging ability and restore it to its natural strength and potency.

You'll find the exercises more useful if you keep the following suggestions in mind.

Concentrate

Distractions inhibit and weaken images. As your skills become renewed and revitalized, you'll be able to image effectively anywhere, at any time. For now, though, try to focus on imagery only in a quiet place where you won't be interrupted.

Pay Attention to Details

You are unique. Specific, concrete details of an image will belong to you alone; they will have meaning for only you. Including personalized details in your imagery will help your mind communicate with your body.

Assign a Logical Sequence to the Image

All your images should make sense to you. Don't ask your mind to image the taste of a banana until you image peeling the banana.

Use All Your Sensors

Probably the most difficult part of remembering how to image well is relearning to take advantage of all our sensors. In this age of television, we tend to rely too much on visual stimuli. But if we trust only our eyes, we deprive ourselves of the smells, tastes, textures, and sounds that all our sensors working together can experience. Remember that imagery is our central sensory processor. It functions regardless of which sensory experiences are available, but it works much better if all sensors contribute. Seeing is indeed an important element in the imaging process, but as we've said before, integrating sound, odor, taste, and touch deepens and expands the mind's understanding of an experience. For imagery to be effective, it must approximate real life as closely as possible. And real life is the product of the input we receive from all our sensors.

SENSORY DEPRIVATION EXERCISES

The first step to learning imagery, therefore, is for you to acquire a greater appreciation of how each sensor adds a unique perspective to your environment and to stop playing favorites. Those of us who are vision dominant, for example, tend to lose sight of the full spectrum of sound all around us. We see the lush green of the grass beneath our feet, but seldom do we listen to the crisp crackle of the leaves in our path.

Perhaps by temporarily blocking out each of the sensors you take for granted, you'll develop a greater respect for their capabilities. Like the song says, "You don't know what you've got 'til it's gone."

The following exercise will be a bit uncomfortable at first, but it is well worth the effort.

EXERCISE ONE: SMELL AND TASTE

Before you sit down to a meal, plug up your nose. You might use your swimming nose plug, or you might want to simply hold your nose.

Now concentrate on how your experience of the

meal changes. You can't smell the food placed before you. How can you use your other sensors to appreciate the meal? Think carefully about what each of your remaining sensors tells you. Does food look different when you can't smell it? Do the sounds around the dinner table carry more meaning?

Place a morsel of food in your mouth. You can't taste it as well as you can without the nose plugs, can you? Think about the texture of the food. Is it stringy or smooth? Tender or tough? Mushy or chunky? How does it feel on your tongue? How does it sound as you chew?

What sensations does it send through your tongue, your mouth, and through your entire body? How do you react to icy cold, or boiling hot? How does bland or spicy feel?

As you swallow, feel how the nutrition spreads through your body. Do you sense your insides warming? What does "full" feel like?

All the way through the meal, concentrate on things your sensors tell you and the ways they compensate for your disabled senses of taste and smell.

EXERCISE TWO: TOUCH

Put on a pair of thick gloves. Then concentrate on the difficulties the bulky gloves cause as you try to do simple tasks.

For example, you might pick up a piece of fruit.

You can't feel its skin. You can't tell whether it's smooth or rough, soft or firm, warm or cool. Does that make it less—or more—appetizing? Bite into it. Does it taste different when you can't feel it?

Hug a child. You can't feel the softness of the child's skin, you can't sense the warmth of his or her body. Do you feel vulnerable, missing these sensations? Do you compensate by listening more closely to the child's words, or breathing? Do you look at the child more intently? Do you smell the shampoo in the hair or the gum the child is chewing?

Wear the gloves while you do some routine tasks. You might choose to wear them while cleaning the house, balancing your checkbook, or eating dinner, for example.

How does your impaired sense of touch affect the way you do things? What sensations are you missing because you can't feel things properly? Are you more aware of your other sensors? Think about how your other sensors help you overcome your handicap.

EXERCISE THREE: HEARING

Plug up your ears. Now go to some familiar place, such as a park or a busy intersection.

After a minute or two, do you see the trees and the flowers in the park more distinctly? Do you feel the cool breeze on your face more intensely? Does the smell of the blossoms seem sweeter? Does nature seem more alive? What do you notice that you never noticed before?

At a busy intersection, are you more aware of the people and vehicles bustling around you? Does the rumble of the trucks passing by seem more ominous? Do the diesel fumes seem more acrid? Think about how vulnerable you feel, out on a crowded street, deprived of your hearing. Notice how keenly you are aware of your other sensors.

Go about some routine tasks. How does the lack of hearing affect how you do things? Concentrate on how the lack of hearing changes even ordinary experiences.

EXERCISE FOUR: SIGHT

Now put on a blindfold. Try to catalog the many ways you can still experience the world without sight.

Sit in your favorite chair. Does it feel different when you can't see what is around you? Can you relax as easily?

What can you hear that you've never really noticed before? The sound of the heater fan or air conditioning? The rush of traffic outside? The creaking of the floor boards?

Do you smell the dust in the air, or the clinging odors left by tonight's pot roast, or the funky smell coming from your socks?

Do you feel the house shudder against the wind? Can you sense someone padding down the hallway in bare feet?

Wear the blindfold in your yard, or in a park. What does sunshine feel like? What does grass smell like? Can you hear the birds flying above?

Experience other common events blindfolded. What does a television program sound like? What does a hug feel like? Does food taste different when you can't see it?

Concentrate on understanding the information your other sensors provide you to overcome your blindness.

Now that you have all your sensors back, we hope you appreciate them more. Specifically, we hope you realize the many ways your sensors work together to help you interpret your experiences. You will need to call on all your sensors to create vivid images. The exercises you have just completed and the ones that follow are intended to help you sharpen your sensors and then fine-tune your imagery. They are important preparatory steps in the process that will, later, allow you to control your imagery well enough to reduce your pain.

Here's one piece of advice: keep in mind the difference between the unfettered freedom of raw imagination and the focused power of imagery. The fantasies, daydreams, and other whimsy sparked by an active imagination are wonderful holidays for your mind. With your imagination you create a special haven that is free from unbalanced checkbooks and dirty laundry. It is a place where you can fly, or win the Olympic finals in the 400-meter hurdles, or address the U.S. Supreme Court.

In contrast, the imagery skills you are learning here require a much clearer and more focused intent.

You are not, however, ready to practice clinical imagery yet. The exercises in this chapter are conditioning exercises, designed to help you reestablish contact with the intuitive and creative parts of your mind—the parts that form the foundation of effective imagery. Think of these exercises as an essential warm-up for using imagery well, similar to the stretching routines and wind sprints of baseball's spring training.

As you go along, you will practice using individual sensors and making them work together. Then you will learn how to use all your sensors in more advanced ways.

EFFECTIVE IMAGERY EXERCISES

EXERCISE ONE

Image an apple sitting in a basket in the center of a table. Make it a table that you are used to sitting at, and make it a kind of apple you've eaten before. The apple has a stem sticking out of it. You reach out and twist the stem, turn it round and round, until you hear it snap off. What did that stem sound like when you pulled it out?

Pick up the apple and hold it in your hand. Your

fingers curl up around the shiny skin. Feel the skin with your fingertips. How does it feel? Hold the apple up to the light coming in from a window. How does the light change the color of the apple? Look at the light reflected on the apple's skin.

Bring the apple up toward your mouth. You're going to eat the apple now. Maybe your mouth begins to water, saliva flowing under your tongue in anticipation. Bite into the apple. Hear the sound as your teeth break through the apple's flesh and sink into the pale pulp. Taste the apple, and inhale its fragrance. Chew. Feel the apple being ground into mush by your teeth. Feel the juice run down your throat. Swallow. Look at the apple again—at the difference between the color of the skin and the gold-white glow of its exposed pulp.

Now repeat the process with a real apple. Feel its skin. Look at its colors. Take a bite and chew it slowly.

How did your image compare to the actual experience of eating an apple?

To help you evaluate the strength of your imaging, we have provided an Imagery Effectiveness Scale. Use this scale to evaluate your image of the apple. Remember what eating a real apple was like. Use that as the benchmark for deciding if aspects of your imaging can be classified as "extremely vivid." Keep in mind, however, that the scale isn't a definitive measure of your imaging skill. It is simply a guide to assist you in adjusting and refining your imagery ability.

IMAGERY EFFECTIVENESS SCALE

Use this scale to evaluate your imaging. Simply choose the number that best describes your experience of each aspect of the image.

Not vivid at all		Average			Extremely vivid

How vivid was what you saw (color, shape, size, etc.)?

0	1	2	3	4	5	6

How vivid was the sound of the image?

0	1	2	3	4	5	6

How vivid was the taste in the image (sweet, sour, salty, etc.)?

0	1	2	3	4	5	6

How vivid was the smell in the image?

0	1	2	3	4	5	6

How vivid was the texture in the image (rough, smooth, etc.)?

0	1	2	3	4	5	6

How vivid was the image?

0	1	2	3	4	5	6

Your total score is the sum of all the individual ratings. If your score is above 30, than your imaging was excellent; 20–29 means your imaging was good.

As you continue through these exercises, you might not feel like evaluating all your images, and you don't have to. Use the scale as a training aid, especially if you think you're having trouble creating clear, effective images.

Here's one point to remember as you proceed. Focusing the mind is important for your imagery. But you have to focus gently, as if adjusting the telephoto lens of a sensitive camera.

Your mind will piece together all the essential elements of your images, but at its own speed. It's better for you to just relax, breathe easily, and let your images evolve naturally.

EXERCISE TWO

Four basic elements make the visual component of images vivid: size, color, depth, and motion. Try to incorporate these elements in your imaging in this exercise.

Think of a door. You walk through the door into a room and step onto the floor. The floor is covered with white and black tiles in a checkerboard pattern.

In the middle of the room is a white tile. On that tile is a big blue glass marble. Image that you're looking at it through the zoom lens of a video or movie camera. Zoom in on the blue marble until it seems to fill your entire mind. All you see is the blue, bright and clear where the light flows through the glass, dark where the light doesn't penetrate.

Slowly zoom out now until the marble is just a speck in the checkerboard pattern of the floor.

Zoom in again and the blue marble seems to be the entire world. Zoom out again and see the marble, as you saw it originally, on the tile floor. Zoom in, then out. Zoom in and out several times.

Add more motion to the image. Move your eyes around the edge of the blue marble. Circle the marble with your eyes a few times; then reverse and go back around the marble a few times. Circle the marble again and again, going faster and faster until the marble seems to be spinning around, moving toward you.

Walk forward onto the next square of the floor and try it again. Keep spinning the marble until you're tired. Then rest.

EXERCISE THREE

This exercise is designed to help you with the tactile aspects of imagery. Have someone put a variety of small objects in a bag, a box, or any container that prevents you from seeing what's inside.

Close your eyes. Now reach in and pull out an object. Keep your eyes closed. Feel what the object looks like. Feel its shape, size, texture, temperature. Explore the entire surface of the object. Image in your mind what the object looks like. Then open your eyes and see how closely your image matches the actual physical appearance of the object.

Repeat this process with each one of the objects in your collection. Use your sense of touch to investigate the objects and let your mind recognize what you discover.

Now try the exercise again. This time have someone select for you objects that are more difficult to identify—objects with irregular shapes, unusual textures, or undifferentiated surfaces. "Read" these objects with your fingers. Image in your mind what the objects look like. Try to determine what they are made of. Guess what is inside them. Create as complete an image as you can.

Choose one of your favorite songs. It might be a current top-ten hit or a golden oldie or a classical masterpiece. As long as it's a song you know well, and one you have a recording of.

Perform the song in your mind. Experience every part of the piece. Play the melody and the harmony. Become the lead vocalist and the backup singers. Hear every individual instrument. Keep time with the rhythm section. Notice every nuance, the subtle pauses, the crescendos, the shrill high notes, the pounding of the bass, even the flubs and the occasional off-key notes.

Then play the actual recording of the song. Use the

Imagery Effectiveness Scale to judge how close your imaged performance comes to the real thing.

EXERCISE FIVE

Here's an exercise to help you integrate the imaginal information gathered by your sensors.

Think of a box. It can be any kind of box, whatever comes to mind. It could be a box of baking soda, or a box of corn flakes, or a box of Tide. It doesn't matter. The box can be any size, any shape.

Lift the box up in your mind. Turn it over. Turn it upside down and hear whatever's inside rattle and slide and settle again. And feel the contents as it hits the sides of the box when it tumbles, feel it move beneath your hand. Shake the box or put it down. Feel the fibrous cardboard in your hand. Look at every side of the box—front, back, sides, top, and bottom. Each surface has colors and letters or numbers. Try to image these in your mind. Try to remember what you've experienced before. That will help you create your image.

How are you doing? If these exercises are somewhat frustrating, don't be discouraged. You were a terrific imager at the age of eight, and practice will help you regain your former prowess. And though it may be tempting to just read through these exercises in your hurry to gain relief from your pain, it is very important for you to actually do all the exercises until you become comfortable with your imaging abilities.

It's time to ease your imaginal ability into second gear. The next series of exercises expands the basic skills we just worked on. Remember to stay relaxed. Don't force images. You don't have to; just sit back and simply let them come, because they always do. Keep your mind clear and undistracted and your body calm.

At the end of each practice session, remember what you felt with each of your sensors. Use the Imagery Effectiveness Scale to critique your performance. Repeat each exercise until you can score in the 28–30 range. Be honest in your self-evaluation. If you don't think you're doing well, review the principles of effective imagery at the beginning of the chapter and try again.

The next two exercises will help you sharpen your ability to image color, depth, and spatial integration.

EXERCISE SIX

Relax and close your eyes. You are surrounded by blackness, swallowed up by peaceful darkness. Image a bright dot of red light far off in the distance. Make the dot grow larger and larger as it comes slowly toward you. Here it comes, closer and closer.

Before the red light reaches you, it begins to pale, fading gradually from scarlet to rose, then pink, then nearly white, until it disappears altogether.

Go over this process again and again, slowly, until you can image the dot, its approach and color change, as if it were right there in front of you.

Off in the black distance, another bright dot of light appears. This one is orange. Think of the orange light moving closer and closer, expanding as it floats toward you. Then the bright orange glow begins to fade, growing pale and softer until it vaporizes, becoming a misty cloud before it disappears.

In the darkness you see a pinpoint of bright yellow light, far away like a miniature sun. It comes toward you, growing larger and brighter, becoming a warm golden circle. Bask in the brightness and warmth of the light. Then the yellow begins to fade, first flaxen, then paler and paler until the light disappears.

There's a clear green dot of light in the darkness, bright and clear like an emerald. Watch it move closer and closer. The clear green light expands until it envelops you in its waves of green. Then watch the green light get paler and softer as it slowly fades and disappears.

You see a soft pale dot of blue light in the distance. Watch this gentle light as it floats closer, a bubble of light, growing large enough to surround and embrace your entire body. The blue light lifts you gently up into the air. The pale color of the light changes as you rise, and you find yourself floating on a cloud of white and luminous light, like the clouds you see from an airplane window.

Feel yourself drifting up into the sky. Look at those

other clouds as you float past them. The clouds are a tranquil place to be, floating peacefully above the earth.

Float for as long as you like. When it's time to come back, return slowly and gently. Drift back into the darkness and stand on your feet again, back on firm ground. Take a deep breath; let the air fill your lungs.

EXERCISE SEVEN

Close your eyes and relax. Think of a red ball, floating in a blue sky. Change the color of the ball. Change it to orange and then to yellow. Move the ball from left to right, up and down; move the ball from side to side, back and forth. Bounce the ball all across the bright blue sky.

Bring the ball closer to you. Then send it spinning away toward the horizon. Make the ball fly so far away you can't see it anymore. Then make it fly back toward you.

Make the ball turn into a balloon, then into a kite. Change the kite into a bird, flying around you until you change it back into a ball again. Now, give up control of the image. Let your mind take the ball and do whatever it wants to with it.

Take control of the ball again. Bounce the ball through the bright sky. When you're ready to stop, open your eyes and restart your conscious mind.

*   *   *

In the next two exercises, you will use real objects and your imagination to sharpen your perception of details.

<u>*EXERCISE EiGHT*</u>

You will practice concentration and attention to detail in this exercise. Start with the objects we suggest, and then move on to objects of your own choice. But choose things that interest you and make you curious.

A. Pick up a rock and hold it in your hand.   Feel its surface. Turn the rock over and over in your hands and feel the texture of the rock, rough or smooth against your skin. Use your fingers to explore every crack, ridge, or crevice on the rock's surface. Is the rock hard or porous or brittle?

Imagine now that you are very small, small enough to crawl on the rock. What do you see? Crawl into a crack and look around. Reach out and touch the rock's interior. Hear the sound of your feet on the rock as you climb around.

Now imagine that you are the rock. How do you feel? Are you heavy or light, large or small? Imagine that you are lying in a field. Tall grass sways above you in the wind. A gentle rain splashes on you from a cloudy sky. How does the rain feel on your rock skin? How does the ground beneath you feel?

Now the rain has stopped, and you notice the clouds moving away. The sun appears. Feel the light from the sun shining down onto your wet rock shell. Smell the grass around you, and the wet ground. Smell yourself, damp from the rain.

Imagine now that you are breaking out of the rock, like a sprout from a seed, growing until you reach your original size.

B. Hold an orange in your hand. Turn it over and over. Toss it up in the air and catch it. Feel its weight. Maybe it's cold. Maybe not. Smell the orange. Lick its skin. Let the fragrance and taste of the skin help you remember what an orange is like when you eat it. Dig your fingernail into the orange's skin and feel some juice spray out onto your hand. Smell the fragrance; isn't it stronger now?

Imagine that you are becoming smaller and smaller, small enough to crawl inside the crease you made with your fingernail in the orange's skin. What does the inside of the orange look like? The color of the orange on the inside is different from the color on the outside, isn't it? Be careful as you walk around inside the orange, so the juice doesn't soak you. What does the orange feel like? Is the fragrance different from what you smelled before?

Taste the orange. Does it make your lips pucker, or is it refreshing, or dry and tasteless?

Imagine that you are the orange, sitting in a plastic net bag in a grocery store. Feel the weight of the other oranges in the bag as they press down on you. You're surrounded by oranges, all imprisoned in the same kind of plastic bags. Smell all the smells of the rest of the produce section. Imagine that someone has picked up the bag of oranges that you are in. You're bumping along in a shopping cart now, rattling past the deli counter and the meat section. See the aisles of the store as they slip past you, a blur of colors and brand names and special offers. See the colors, and hear the cart rattle, and the other carts too.

Feel the temperature change as you move down the frozen food aisle in your cart. If they put that ice cream any closer to you in the cart, you'll be a frozen orange.

Feel yourself being packed into a paper bag. Feel the canned goods pressing down on you and feel yourself pressing against the other oranges in the bag. Now you're in a car, but you can't see anything; the sounds of the street are barely audible from inside the trunk. Now you're in the air again; you'll be inside the house soon. Feel the temperature of the air outside, and smell the air—clean, a welcome change from the fumes inside the trunk.

Inside the house, you and the other oranges are set free from the plastic net bag. You roll and tumble into a basket. Now you feel the basket being lifted up, and you come to rest, finally, in the refrigerator, near the cheese.

Leave the orange's interior now, and come back to

the room you're in, back to your normal size. Try to remember everything you saw, smelled, heard, felt, and tasted as an orange.

C. Sit down on a carpet somewhere where you will be comfortable. Feel the carpet. Let your hands wander over it. If the carpet is thick enough, push your hands down into the pile and run your hands through the fibers. Feel the fibers tangled between your fingers. Feel the texture of the rough carpet against your skin.

Imagine that you are getting smaller and smaller, until you are small enough to stroll between the fibers of the carpet. Take a walk in the carpet. Kick that crumb out of the way. (It looks like a boulder but it's bread.) Hear the sound the carpet fibers make when you brush against them.

Look up and see the room from down where you are. Imagine that you are melting into the carpet—you are becoming part of the carpet, a fiber, standing up next to other carpet fibers, tough but flexible.

What's it like to be part of a carpet? See someone coming. Shoes look different from underneath, don't they? And they smell like the damp ground outside; it must be raining. What did it sound like when that shoe pushed all those fibers against each other and against you too? Were you flattened? How long did it take to spring back?

Imagine that you are growing, getting larger and larger like a stalk of wheat. Now you're back to your original size. But don't forget what it was like to be a carpet fiber—the smells, the feelings, the sounds.

Here are some other objects that you might find useful for this exercise: a plant, an ice cube, a ball of string, a bowl of Jello, a can of soda. Be creative. Think of your own objects and use the same exploratory process to examine them. Remember as many of the imagined and imaged feelings as you can. Become accustomed to sensory details; this focused attention will help you later.

<hr>

EXERCISE NINE

In the last exercise, you sharpened your awareness of details. Now you will examine how details make you feel.

Make a list of objects found in and around your home. Choose objects of all different sizes and shapes. We have provided a list of examples to get you started, but you can surely think of many more. Be as creative as you can.

The lamp in your living room.
A car.
The cover of this book.
Your favorite chair.
Your house keys.
A pen.

A garden hose.

A bowling ball.

A steam iron.

Your television set.

A particular tree.

A diamond ring.

Your alarm clock.

A loaf of bread.

A pair of shoes.

A telephone.

A refrigerator.

A toothbrush.

Pick an object, and image how you react to it. For example, if you image your car, you might see the gleam of its shine, smell the odor of the leather upholstery, feel the surge of its acceleration, and hear the throaty rumble of its exhaust. You also might experience the anxiety of merging onto a crowded freeway, or the exhilaration of powering through a hairpin turn. Think of as many details as you can, and image how you react to each detail.

Choose about ten objects, and image how you react to each item. Make your images as complete as you can.

The next two exercises help you involve your memory in the imaging process.

Memory is a valuable tool in imagery. Our minds

have trouble understanding abstract concepts like "peace," "happiness," or "love." But our unconscious can guide us to our experiences of these feelings through imagery selected from impressions of the past. Your mind recognizes "happiness" only when your imagery reproduces a sensory representation of the feelings you associate with happiness. Years ago, a book claimed that happiness was "a warm puppy." Corny perhaps, but from an imaginal perspective, completely valid.

EXERCISE TEN

Think of a place where you once lived, a place you associate with pleasant memories. Remember the street where you lived? What was it like? See your house now, as you walk down your old street. Hear the noises you used to hear when you walked down that street. The cars, the giggling kids, your neighbor's weed whacker, barking dogs—let it all come back.

You're outside your home. Can you see it? Go to the front door, hear it open, and then hear it close behind you. Walk into the living room and sit down. Touch the things you see. Pick them up. Feel the weight and shape and textures of the objects you find.

Think of the way the house used to smell. Food

cooking, hairspray, aftershave, your pets, furniture polish, laundry detergent. Remember the sounds of the rooms: music, laughter, talking, or the banging of the radiator pipes and the creaking of the walls.

Go into all the rooms and stay as long as you like. Remember as much as you can, in as much detail as you can muster.

Relive a happy childhood experience. Maybe it's a special Christmas, or a trip to the Ice Capades. Maybe you went to the circus, or you got to see the mighty Ted Williams put one over the right-field wall in Boston. A fishing trip with your father, perhaps, or your best birthday party. A school dance, where you discovered that he or she liked you too. Your first fumble in the back seat of a car. It can be anything you want.

Feel what you felt then. Feel and hear and taste and smell and see what your sensors were sensing then. Concentrate and think of as many details as you can.

How are you doing? This next set of exercises will help you reacquaint yourself with the creative aspects of your imagery skills. A strong internal focus plays a major role in these exercises. We'll set the scene, but then you take it wherever you want from there. Use your memories to create images.

EXERCISE TWELVE

You are walking down a hallway. On your left is a blank solid wall, stretching down a long, empty corridor. On your right are windows covered by billowing gauze curtains. Walk down the hall, with the curtains blowing and twisting in front of you and behind you, until you come to a door.

Open the door.

What's on the other side?

EXERCISE THIRTEEN

You are walking in a forest. The sky is blue. A canopy of green leaves and twisted branches is stretched out over your head. The air is fresh—it tastes clean when it hits your throat. Feel the wind—it's light, and it's rustling the leaves above you.

You lean up against a tree for a while and watch the birds fly from branch to branch. Watch the squirrels chase each other, bounding down from the trunk of a tree. When you feel like it, continue your walk.

You push through some low-hanging branches and

you find yourself on an old dirt road. Walk down the road.

Where does it go?

EXERCISE FOURTEEN

This is the final exercise. Here you will combine the skills you have practiced in the previous exercises to create a vivid, extended image. With this exercise, you will see how you can use your imaging skills to relax your mind and your body.

Image yourself lying back in a small boat. You have thick, soft cushions tucked under you and lying around you. You feel comfortable and safe. Your boat is floating down a narrow channel. The sun is filtering through the leaves in the tops of the oak trees that arch above you. You see the shadows of the leaves flickering on your body.

Underneath you, you feel the gentle rocking of the boat as you float along on the current. Water slaps softly against the sides of your boat. It's early summer; so it's warm but not sticky or humid. You float downstream. Smell the forest smells, and the smells of the waterway. Let all your sensors investigate the world around you.

Look over the side of the boat. See the fish swimming in the stream. Notice their color and their shapes as they dart back and forth under the water and under the boat. They look as if they're being reflected in a fun house mirror, distorted by the moving water. Let your hand trail in the stream. Feel the refreshing coolness of the water.

Splash some water on your face. Look around you at the banks of the stream. What do you see? Try to remember everything. Look up at the sky. Be aware of everything around you. Relax. Feel content and serene as you drift on.

You're coming up to a tunnel now, but you've been through this tunnel before, so you know what to expect. Darkness, then escape. A good place for shade when it's hot. As you float into the tunnel, you can't see anything except the sunlight sparkling on the water at the other end. Your boat is drifting slowly into the darkness, and your mind wanders. Where does it go? It's always moving, into the past, back into the present, probing into the future. Linger in the tunnel, dream in the tunnel, for as long as you want.

As you come out of the tunnel, you feel yourself being covered by golden sunshine. The sunlight wraps itself around you and brings you energy and makes you smile. You glide out of the tunnel and come to a lake.

You float out onto the lake. A cool breeze sweeps across your body. The lake is tranquil. Nearly silent. Feel the quiet.

Be aware of everything: the gentle motion of the

boat, the warmth of the sun, the fragrances (there's lavender growing somewhere along the lake), the sounds of just drifting along. Let yourself feel these sensations.

You're floating on the lake, your little boat circling like a satellite, not going anywhere else. This lake is where you want to be.

Come back from this exercise slowly. Reacquaint yourself with where you really are sitting. Open your eyes and look around the room.

How do you feel?

We hope this last exercise has relaxed you, but we realize that most of the imaging you have just done can be exhausting work. And that's to be expected. After all, this is exercise, and it can be as tiring as lifting weights. Just as a beginning weight lifter must condition and develop unused or underused muscles, you must condition and develop unused or underused sensors.

As you progress through these exercises, however, you gain imaginal fitness. You build up your ability to use all your sensors to create vivid, lifelike images. This imaginal fitness will be central to the pain-control process that is to come.

We can't predict how much practice you'll need to master the basic imagery skills you've been working on in this chapter. Keep practicing until you are comfortable with the process of feeling and sensing as much as you can, in your mind and with your body. Don't lose heart if your performance disappoints you. Some people need more time to awaken their sense of imagery from its long rest. Use the principles of effective imagery and the Imagery Effectiveness Scale as training aids, but don't worry too much about them or the mechanics of imagery. Rest easy and keep imaging. Your mind and body will recognize what you are trying to communicate if you simply concentrate and let it happen.

CHAPTER 7

Zeroing In:
Pain-Control Imagery

> *Pain is where it hurts.*
> —CHARLIE BROWN,
> "PEANUTS"

By now, you should be comfortable with your imagery skills. You should be able to create clear, realistic images quickly and easily. The exercises you have completed—if you've done them seriously and diligently—have shown you how to shape and focus your images. The next step, the vital advance, is to learn to create images you can use to control your pain.

You begin with the experience of pain. Then, you interpret the pain, seeking images and terms that your mind's apparatus can recognize. Next, you develop an autogenic prompt—a powerful image your

mind can use to attack your pain. Finally, you use
this prompt and your imagery skills to overcome, or
escape from, your pain.

PAIN-CONTROL IMAGERY
The experience of pain
↓
The interpretation of pain
↓
The autogenic prompt
↓
Control of pain

The key to this formula is the prompt. By developing a powerful image to counter your pain, you
create a force that your mind—and then your body—
can respond to. If you work diligently to make the
prompt a fixed image you can call upon at will, this
control image will become an autogenic prompt—a
self-generated, specially coded message that can deal
with your pain. "Autogenic" means self-generated
or self-produced. Making your prompt autogenic involves a synthesis of the imagery skills you have
been working on. With practice, the small steps you
have learned will become a great leap. They will become a conditioned response. Merely calling upon
your prompt will bring about the desired result. In
other words, you condition yourself to feel better in
response to your prompt. You might even think of

your prompt as a form of therapy you can keep in your pocket and pull out whenever you need it.

After you practice imaging and develop an effective prompt, control of your chronic pain can become as spontaneous and automatic as the control you now exert over voluntary physical functions. It can be as simple as taking a step, or raising your hand, or just saying "stop hurting."

To give you an idea of how simply it can work, here's one case history reported by Gary Schwartz of Yale University, who has written extensively on imagery in pain control. Several years ago, a three-year-old boy who suffered severe migraine headaches was treated at the Yale Behavioral Medicine Clinic. His therapists knew that a major cause of the migraines was too much blood rushing through the arteries in the boy's head. They reasoned that the migraines could be alleviated by redirecting the flow of blood. They decided to teach the boy to use imagery to make his hands feel warm, hoping that would channel the flow of blood to his fingers and thereby lessen the severity of the migraines. The boy was told to image "hot thoughts" in order to warm his hands.

The procedure worked. But the therapists were amazed when the boy went one step further on his own. He figured out a way to compress the imagery technique into a verbal command. By simply saying out loud, "Hands, you're hot," the boy could raise the temperature on his hands by ten to fifteen degrees. For this boy, the phrase "Hands, your hot" had become an autogenic prompt. Schwartz estimated that the boy's deceptively simple prompt actually involved the "integration of nine major levels of social psychoneurophysiological processes."

We have found that imagery, while immeasurably complicated in its actual operation, is really quite simple when approached from a pragmatic point of view. Other pain-management professionals who have analyzed guided imagery have classified, categorized, and subdivided imaginal control techniques into dozens of technical pigeonholes. We feel no need to be that pedantic. Our experience has shown us that people respond to imagery in two basic ways. Some people respond to abstract concepts. Others respond to empirical data. On the basis of that division, we have identified two distinct types of clinical imagery that can be used for practical pain-control purposes. We call them subjective imagery and objective imagery. We are confident *all* pain sufferers can use one of these two types of imagery.

Each style of imagery involves its own process, and each has proven to be effective for different types of people. During our research we have discovered that some people can accurately describe their experience of pain by using symbols. They say, for example, that the pain in their chest feels like a ton of bricks pressing down on them, or their headache makes their head pound like a drum. For these people, subjective imagery generally works.

Others can relate to their pain only in prosaic terms. They view chest pain as a pain in their chest; a headache is an aching in the head. As Charlie Brown says, "Pain is where it hurts." For them, objective imagery based on physiology works.

The simple fact is that different people respond to different types of imagery. Some people are more intuitive, and others are more literal (in fact, some people with neurological damage are actually incapable of thinking clearly in the abstract). Either way, however, clinical imagery can be used to attack pain.

Let's take a closer look at the two forms of clinical imagery. Later you can try each approach and determine which works best for you.

SUBJECTIVE IMAGERY

The method of subjective imagery starts, of course, with the experience of pain. Your head hurts, your back aches, or you have a pain in your chest. Knowing where your pain is located, however, is not sufficient. With subjective imagery, the important fact is not where you hurt; it's how the pain makes you feel.

First, you creatively interpret your pain by using a symbolic impression—an image that clearly communicates what your pain feels like to your sensors. This usually can be achieved without a great deal of effort. What hurts? "My back hurts." What does it feel like? "It feels as if someone's driving a sharp spike into my spinal cord."

To gain control of the pain, you must develop an autogenic prompt, an image you can call upon as a defense to help you lessen your pain, or in some cases, cause the pain to subside completely. If your image of pain is a sharp spike being driven into your spinal cord, for example, your prompt might be an image of strong hands pulling that spike out. Developing the autogenic prompt is crucial. Work and practice and more work and more practice are usually required before your mind will connect the image of pain with the image of an effective defense.

At first, it might seem obvious that someone in pain should know all too well what his or her pain feels like. Yet most people are used to experiencing pain, not interpreting it. It's difficult to think straight when you're in pain and it's easy to be overwhelmed by your suffering to the exclusion of all else. However, if your pain can be characterized, it can be dealt with.

In the Guide to Subjective Imagery we've given you examples of words and images that are often used to interpret chronic pain. You may find a word or phrase that describes what your pain feels like on the list. If not, don't worry. You suffered with your pain long before we came along. You know it well. Subjective imagery takes its name from the fact that your image of your pain is yours alone.

Look at the list, and use it as a guide. Consider the

GUIDE TO SUBJECTIVE IMAGERY

Experience	Interpretation	Autogenic Prompt
biting	vicious dogs	muzzles
burning	searing flames	cool water spray
crushing	vise	metal bar to jam vise
grinding	rusty gears	oil/lubricant
stabbing	sharp knife	armor
heaviness	stack of bricks	hoist/pulley
numbness	ice	heating pad/hot pack
piercing	sword	shield
pounding	bass drum	thick cotton to muffle impact
throbbing	blood pulsing	valve on vein to slow blood flow
squeezing	clenched fist	uncurl hand one finger at a time

connection that is made between the pain and the counteracting prompt in addition to the words and the images themselves. If an image from the list strikes a familiar chord, use it. It's still your subjective image. What you think of when you image a knife plunged into your back will always be different from someone else's experience of the same image. That's the way we are, infinitely variable and individually unique. Most important of all, be creative as you consider images. Use the techniques you studied in Chapter 6 to involve all your sensors as you construct images of your pain and its antidote. You may wish to use the Imagery Effectiveness Scale on page 66 to gauge the success of your imagery.

Always be specific with your image of pain. If "hot" is the primary sensation you associate with your pain, decide what "hot" means to you. Is it a suffocating and constant heat like a blast from an oven? Or is it the sharp, focused heat like the heat generated by the glowing red point of a hot poker?

At first, it might be difficult to be clear about your experience of pain. We tend to think of pain as pain. If you have had months or years of lower back pain, you may by now think of it only as "your pain." People don't often refer to their back pain as "my hot sensation" or "my throbbing back." We tend to say "my back hurts," and we continue to suffer. But in your mind, in the area where all your sensory experiences are stored, there is an exactly right way for you to image what your pain feels like. To use subjective imagery, you must be able to give your pain a specific description. That description, your description of your pain, is the key to the selection of an effective prompt and, eventually, relief from your chronic pain.

The following case history will clarify our point. It's the story of a patient of ours who had horrible migraine headaches every few weeks. The pain wasn't constant, she said, but it was bad enough and frequent enough to make her life miserable.

When her pain attacked, she became dizzy and

nauseated. She felt as if she were being crushed by a tremendous pressure. She said her pain felt like a vise squeezing the left side of her skull. Each time one of her headaches struck, the vise seemed to press tighter and tighter, compressing the inside of her head so viciously that she couldn't lift her head off her pillow. She felt that her only recourse was to lie still and pray for the pain to go away.

We were pleased that the woman was able to describe her pain with something as specific as a vise. The vise was a clear, if unfortunate, image that we (and she) could use in her defense. We suggested that the woman image a metal bar, a solid, unbendable, unbreakable metal bar specially tempered to withstand the pressure of the vise. We asked her to insert the bar into the vise, and to pry the vise open and keep it from squeezing during the migraine attacks.

The point is that the vise, a symbolic representation of pain, helped the woman create a counteracting prompt, the metal bar. The image of the metal bar inserted in the vise to keep it from clamping down helped the woman control her pain.

When she had thoroughly mastered the imagery process, the woman no longer had to specifically image the vise. She didn't have to remind herself that the bar was stronger than the vise. All she had to do was image the metal bar and her mind completed the connection.

Another patient came to us with Reynaud's syndrome. People with Reynaud's have poor circulation that results in painfully cold fingers, hands, toes, and feet.

We suggested that she image her hands being put into thick electric gloves, like electric blankets with fingers. We asked her to image the gloves becoming so hot that she would have to take them off soon after putting them on, to avoid burning her hands.

We also asked her to image special electric socks that would warm her feet.

After some practice, the woman was able to image the gloves and socks to generate warmth in her hands and feet, and she was more comfortable.

You can see that once an experience of pain is put into symbolic (imaginal) terms, an autogenic prompt can be created to help stop the hurting. The steel rod keeps the vise open; the electric gloves and socks warm the cold hands and feet.

As long as you can communicate your pain experience to your mind in such a way that your mind will call upon your autogenic prompt, your pain can be controlled. You don't need to understand the specific cause of your pain—just how it makes you feel. Your mind and nervous systems are sophisticated enough to interpret the message you're sending. That message, stripped to its basics, is simple and direct: *no more pain.*

Another patient came to us with chronic angina or heart pain. This man said that it felt like a load of bricks on his chest, pressing down and pushing his heart back into his spine. His autogenic prompt became a rope and pulley, a hoist that would lift the bricks off his chest. It doesn't matter if someone else thinks that bricks are an odd way to represent pain. All that matters is that to the man in pain, the bricks represent the pain, and the hoist represents relief from that pain. The mind realizes that the ultimate goal is the elimination of the pain, and your internal systems have an astonishing sense of what you're trying to communicate. Imagery is just your way of talking to them. Your mind and body will do what you ask if you communicate your needs effectively. That may seem difficult, but it's not. It can be done. It has been done. You can do it.

OBJECTIVE IMAGERY

Many people cannot interpret their experience of pain in symbols or metaphor. They are unable to articulate—even to themselves—what their pain feels like. "I hurt," they say, and that is truly as specific as they can be.

Subjective imagery is of no use to these individuals. Their minds do not understand or will not accept symbolic messages. Fortunately, a pain-control protocol based upon objective imagery has often been successful when subjective imagery is inappropriate or ineffective.

Objective imagery focuses on the empirical aspects

of your pain. It requires you to examine where you hurt and why you hurt. You must become a detective, searching out objective data about the cause of your pain and its effects. By understanding how your body works and what causes your pain, you can develop an image you can use to deal with your pain.

Objective imagery, like its subjective counterpart, originates with the pain experience. Instead of creating a metaphor for the pain, however, you focus upon the physical site of your pain. Once you isolate the specific source of your pain, the objective-imagery approach will allow you to design an autogenic prompt to counteract that pain. Objective and subjective imagery differ only in the interpretation of the pain. The destination is the same, but the paths are different.

How would you use objective imagery for severe migraines? First, you'd investigate the cause of your pain.

A widely held theory is that migraines are caused by a dilation of the arteries in your head, which allows a great volume of blood to rush through. This typically results in an excruciating pounding or throbbing sensation.

Next, you devise a prompt to stop your pain at its source—perhaps an image of a tiny clip pinching the arteries and slowing down the blood flow in order to reduce the pulsating in your head.

To experiment with objective imagery, talk to your doctor, and ask to see X rays or diagrams of the physical site of your pain. Read all you can about your specific problem. The more completely you know your pain, the better equipped you are in your search for a useful defense. The Guide to Objective Imagery shows the kind of information you'll need and the types of prompts you might create.

Create an image strong enough that you can feel what is happening inside your body as it happens: a joint inflaming, blood vessels constricting or suddenly dilating, torn muscles being twisted or stretched. Study your pain carefully. Turn it over in your mind to feel it with all your sensors, just as you felt objects in the imaging exercises. Then develop a prompt that can counteract the pain: a valve to open blood vessels or close them off, a personalized superglue to mend torn muscles. As with subjective imagery, the specific prompt is up to you. You will need to experiment to find one that responds to your pain.

Here are two more case histories showing how objective imagery works.

One of our patients suffered from severe arthritis in her knees, elbows, and knuckles. Her joints were inflamed and painful, but she could not come up with any specific image of that pain. Instead, she learned all she could about her problem. She talked to her doctors, and she attended lectures to learn about arthritis. Her research told her that the pain and inflammation stemmed from a deterioration in the lining of the joints. She learned specifically that the joints lacked proper lubrication. Armed with that in-

GUIDE TO OBJECTIVE IMAGERY

Experience	Interpretation	Autogenic prompt
arthritis	inflammation of the joints	soothing lubricant
gout	deposits of uric acid crystals in joints	warm water to surround area and dissolve crystals
migraines	sudden vascular dilation: rush of blood to brain	clamp to slow the flow of blood
Reynaud's syndrome	poor circulation to hands and feet	electric gloves and socks to promote warmth and increase circulation
lower back pain	acute ligament (sprain) or muscular (strain) problems	tight wrap around spinal cord for support and to reduce tension
cancer	rapid generation of mutant cell tissue	Pacmen gobbling up mutant cells
spastic colon	excessive production of gastric acid	sponge to soak up acid

formation, she was able to develop an image. She saw herself as the "Tin Lady," like the Tin Man in the *Wizard of Oz*. Then, when pain and inflammation struck, she imaged an oil can squirting lubrication on her stiff joints, just as Dorothy squirted oil to free up the Tin Man's rusted limbs.

Another patient of ours suffered from Reynaud's syndrome, the disorder that causes painfully cold hands and feet. Through his fact-finding, our patient learned that his problem stemmed from poor circulation in his hands and feet. He also learned that warming his extremities would increase the circulation. From those facts he was able to develop an image of hot compresses wrapped around his feet and thick wool gloves covering his hands to increase the circulation. This form of objective imagery brought him significant relief.

You may remember that when we described subjective imagery we told of a woman who suffered from Reynaud's syndrome. She had used imaged gloves and electric blankets to generate warmth. These two patients used similar images, but their minds responded to them in different ways. The woman's prompt focused on the fact her hands and feet felt cold. Her mind responded to the abstract idea of heat warming her cold extremities. The man's prompt focused on his need for better circulation. His mind responded to the concrete physiological reaction. However, the two different interpretations of pain brought similar results—relief.

We have seen both types of imagery—subjective and objective—used often and used effectively. Which is best for you? We don't know, and until you experiment with both, neither do you. There's no test we can give you; only you can find out.

We can only reiterate our message that it's worth your best efforts to master imagery. It's the most powerful self-treatment technique there is, because it's the most direct, and it's the only process that uses a language that both mind and body understand. What we call an autogenic prompt is simply an imaginal message, the biopsychological equivalent of a telegram, a phone call, or a postcard. A simple and honest message will rarely be misunderstood. However, it is essential to choose an image that suits you and truly addresses your pain. Otherwise, the message might not get through. You might be faced with starting the process all over again later.

We can't tell you the specific image that will best control your chronic pain. Ice will cool a fire. Armor will deflect a sword. Movers will lift the piano that sits on your chest. You'll know the best image for you when you feel it.

The representation of your pain and the counteracting image are personal choices, decisions that only you can make. Their effectiveness depends upon your entire lifetime of experience and associations. Only by trying can you find the images that your mind will understand and act upon.

Does it sound too simple? Just identify your pain in terms that the mind understands, create a prompt to counteract the pain, and, through practice and experience, make the control process autogenic.

That's it?

That's all?

Well, yes and no. Running a marathon is relatively easy for marathon runners but torture for weekend joggers. Flying an airplane is automatic if you've been trained for it, incredibly frightening if you haven't. Knowing what to do to control your pain and actually being able to do it are not the same thing.

We want to stress the importance of practicing your imaging skill. As with any new skill, practice and repetition are necessary to make it a natural part of your life. The imagery exercises in Chapter 6 are an important element of your training regimen. Return to those basics whenever you feel your images becoming vague or stale.

Before we take you through the process of using pain-control imagery, however, there is one more issue to consider. You need to prepare your mind and body for the task ahead. You need to put yourself in a state of readiness, a state of mind in which you are most receptive to change. The way to achieve this state is through total relaxation. Once you have learned effective relaxation techniques, your chances for success will be greatly increased.

CHAPTER 8

Focusing on Relaxation

Perhaps the concept of relaxation can be introduced best by explaining what it is not. Relaxation is not necessarily lounging in front of the television or playing a leisurely round of golf. Contrary to widespread opinion, being relaxed does not mean just being sedentary or getting away from the job. If you're watching TV and worrying about a project deadline, or if you're playing golf and thinking about the business deal you're trying to close, you're not relaxing at all.

True relaxation is something that is much more calming. It is a process of learning a behavior that unencumbers mind and body, causing a series of healthful physical reactions. When you are relaxed, your heart rate and blood pressure drop. Blood flows to the brain and the skin, rather than to the muscles. Your rate of breathing and your consumption of oxygen decline, and your brain waves shift to a relaxed rhythm. The result is that you feel warm, rested, and mentally alert.

We all need to relax. Specifically, we need to dodge stress. But stress in an unavoidable fact of life. The pressures of work and relationships, the aggravations of our daily routine, and other attacks on our minds and bodies—both real and imagined—are with us every day. As stress builds our heartbeat quickens, blood pressure rises, and our digestive system functions less efficiently. We become more susceptible to a variety of ills. Studies have shown that stress and anxiety can inhibit the functioning of our immune system. Normally, our minds stimulate our bodies to produce an array of chemical antibodies and disease-fighting cells, but stress and anxiety can short-circuit the process. One study of college students found that the production of these disease fighters was inhibited in students facing the pressure and stress of exams, making them much more susceptible to catching colds. Other studies have confirmed that people who are not good at handling stress are more susceptible to disease. There are strong indications that such people may also have less pain tolerance.

True relaxation, the deep, inner peace essential in all mind-based therapies, is a skill that must be learned and practiced. Like imagery, it might seem difficult at first, but with practice you will master it. Over time it can become as easy to use and as autogenic as your prompt.

How? You must concentrate, and learn to focus your mind on the rhythms of your body. You're not relaxing if you're lying on your bed wondering if

you're going to be dragged off to debtor's pris
week because your electric bill is late. "Will 1
get a job I like?" "Will I ever meet the person 1
been waiting for?" Questions like these are to relax
ation what nuclear weapons are to world peace.

The problem is, we're usually so concerned with
our external lives that we don't often examine who
or what we are. Most of us pay more heed to our
conscious, compulsively organized, relentlessly ac-
quisitive outer selves than to the contemplative and
inquisitive side of our nature. Let your external con-
cerns float away. Detach yourself from the world
outside. Until you master relaxation, effective imagery is going to be difficult if not impossible.

In this chapter we will teach you our modified version of the most widely used relaxation techniques.

EFFECTIVE BREATHING

The first step in the relaxation process is learning
to breathe properly. Slow, deep, and regular breathing is essential to relaxation. You may not think of
breathing as something you need to work at, but
most of us do not breathe very efficiently. Most of us
breathe through our mouths instead of our noses.
We breathe too quickly, as if someone were going to
take the air away. And our breathing is too shallow,
involving only our upper chest and throat. But that is
not how we originally learned to breathe. Watching

a baby breathe shows how it should be done. Each time the baby breathes in, the belly rises. When it breathes out, the belly flattens. Each inhalation pushes the diaphragm down, and each exhalation relaxes the entire respiratory system. That is a much more efficient way to breathe. You can take in eight to ten times more oxygen when you breathe this way. Since it provides more effective oxygenization of the blood, proper breathing promotes good health and a good feeling.

The following exercise will help you improve your breathing and increase your body's receptiveness to the relaxation process we'll teach you shortly.

Sit comfortably in a chair, or lie down on a bed, a couch, or the floor. Put your hands on your belly. Close your eyes and breathe in slowly through your nose. Inhale, making your belly expand, not your chest. Feel your belly move out as you draw in the air. Inhale as much air as your lungs can hold. Then try to take in just a bit more. Exhale slowly. Feel your belly move in. When you think you are finished exhaling, try to force out just a little bit more air.

Breathe these deep breaths for a minute or two. Breathe slowly and deeply, from the bottom of your abdomen. This is called belly breathing. If your stomach is moving up and down with your breaths, you're doing fine.

Now, breathe in an easy, regular rhythm, with every inhalation taking the same length of time. It's a bit like dancing. Choose a tempo.

Inhale while you count to four. Hold your breath and count to four. Exhale while you count to four. Then pause and count to four.

Breathe like this:

Inhale	2, 3, 4
Hold	2, 3, 4
Exhale	2, 3, 4
Pause	2, 3, 4

Repeat the series four times.

Now, slow down the tempo:

Inhale	2, 3, 4, 5, 6
Hold	2, 3, 4, 5, 6
Exhale	2, 3, 4, 5, 6
Pause	2, 3, 4, 5, 6

Repeat the series four times.

Find a tempo that feels comfortable to you, and practice using that tempo. There's no right or wrong tempo; you just have to decide what feels good for you.

Once you've mastered deep, regular breathing, you're ready to move on to the next step, detachment.

DETACHMENT

Detachment is the process of releasing your mind from your body, allowing it to float freely and weightlessly.

Learning to achieve detachment is the pivotal point of the relaxation regimen, just as learning your autogenic prompt is the key to the pain-control protocol. It is not easy, but if you follow these steps and work at it, you will succeed.

To begin, make yourself comfortable. Find a place where you won't be disturbed or interrupted. Take the phone off the hook, if necessary. Loosen any tight clothing.

Put yourself in a comfortable posture. Finding the right position is an individual decision, but keep these suggestions in mind.

1. Whether you're sitting or lying down, rest your hands comfortably at your sides. Make sure your muscles are not tensed or flexed. Your legs should be slightly apart, and your toes should be pointed out.

2. Part your lips slightly, and let your tongue rest against your upper teeth, as if you were about to say "la."

Now you are ready to proceed. Begin belly breathing, using an easy, regular cadence. Now, let your body go limp. Let go of all your muscles, making your body feel like just dead weight. To find out how well you are doing, it is helpful to have a partner assist you. When you think you are fully detached, signal your partner by raising a finger. At that point, your partner should raise one of your arms and then release it. The arm should flop to your side, as if it weren't even a part of your body. It should be a good feeling, a feeling of total freedom from the burden of your body.

At first, many people find their arm tenses up when their partner lifts it. It's difficult for us to just let go. But if you keep trying, you should be able to achieve the pleasant freedom of detachment. However, some of you may find it difficult to free yourselves, to go totally limp. If you have trouble fully releasing the tension in your body, you might want to try progressive muscle relaxation. This technique helps you learn how to release tension in each muscle group; one at a time.

With progressive relaxation, you alternately tense and relax the muscles in every part of your body. As we just suggested, start by finding a quiet place and get yourself into a comfortable position. Begin belly breathing in a slow cadence. Now curl your toes as tightly as possible. Keep your toes curled for five seconds. Then, let them uncurl, slowly and completely. (Do you feel the difference?) By systematically tensing and relaxing individual muscles you can become familiar with the difference between tension and relaxation. And you can learn to spread the feeling of relaxation throughout your body.

Start with your toes and work your way up through your feet to your legs, and then your trunk, your chest, shoulders, arms and fists, neck and face. Make yourself as tense as you can, and then just a little bit more tense. Hold that tension as you count slowly from one to five, then relax. Unwind completely. Release all control. Focus on the pleasant feeling of relaxation as it spreads throughout your entire body. Mentally scan your body from head to toe. If you find any muscle that isn't completely relaxed, tighten it, hold the tension for five seconds, then let it go.

Once you have reached a pleasant state of detachment, you are ready to move on to the final step in the relaxation process.

USING IMAGERY TO RELAX

So far you have established a cadence of belly breathing and reached a state of detachment. Now you will use imagery to crowd out unpleasant thoughts and immerse yourself in a state of serenity, security, and comfort.

Begin by thinking of a pleasant image. It might be a place you are fond of or an activity you enjoy. For example, you might image fishing on a clear blue lake, or walking through a luscious garden, or gently rocking a sleeping baby.

Once you have a clear image in mind, close your eyes. Some people are distracted by anxious thoughts when they close their eyes, so repeat to yourself three or four words related to your image. For example, if your image is fishing on a clear blue lake, you might say, over and over, "clear blue lake, clear blue lake. . . ." Repeat the phrase, almost as if it were a mantra. Use it to crowd out any free-floating nega-tive thoughts.

Continue the process for about fifteen minutes. Thirty minutes would be even better. The goal is to train your mind and body to relax. We can't really tell you when you have succeeded. You will be able to tell yourself by answering this simple question: do you feel calm and rested, yet mentally alert?

Remember, your goal is to put your mind and body in a state that is receptive to change. If you learn and practice this relaxation regimen before us-ing pain-control imagery, you will find it easier to learn and the results more rewarding.

CHAPTER 9

A Clear View: Using Your New Control

Now it's time to come out of the shadows and into the sun. Don't be afraid. Everything you've read about and done so far has prepared you for this moment.

You're about to put all the skills you have learned to work. You're about to *do* something about your pain. That might be a scary thought. What if it doesn't work? What if it's just another failed attempt to find relief?

We can only urge you to go ahead. Don't be afraid. It will work. We have seen it work so many times before.

First, let's review the components of pain-control imagery:

> The experience of pain
> The interpretation of pain
> The autogenic prompt
> Control of pain.

Now let's give it a try.

Just as a new driver doesn't charge into rush-hour traffic on the expressway the first time out, it's best at first to try your imagery in a quiet and relatively pain-free environment—not when your pain is at its worst.

Start by using your relaxation regimen. Use belly breathing to establish a slow, regular cadence for your breathing. Let your body go limp and give yourself the pleasant, free-floating feeling of detachment. Use imagery to crowd out unpleasant thoughts and immerse yourself in a state of serenity, security, and comfort.

When you're thoroughly relaxed and comfortable, begin to confront your pain.

First, examine the subjective or objective image you have selected that characterizes your pain. Use all your sensors. Probe all the surfaces, edges, and angles of your pain. See and feel it and try to understand why it makes you hurt. If you are using a subjective image, fully image the source of the pain. Feel the tip of the spike at your spine or feel the vise pressing your skull. If you are using objective imagery, examine the mechanics that are causing your pain. Spend as long as it takes to create a vivid image. It might be two minutes, or it might be fifteen. To start, you might want to expect to spend about ten minutes on this image.

Second, concentrate on your autogenic prompt, the image you have developed to counteract the pain. See and feel it and try to understand how it can relieve your pain. Refine your mental perceptions until every aspect of your image feels just right. The more accurate it feels, the better your body will respond to it. Again, you may wish to spend about ten minutes on your imaging.

Now put the prompt to work.

See and feel your autogenic prompt slowly working on your pain. Image how your pain recedes in response to the action of your prompt as it relieves the cause of the pain. Spend about ten minutes imaging how your prompt counteracts your pain.

Do you feel any better? After your first attempt, maybe not. It may take your mind and body time to absorb what you're trying to tell them. So do it again. Practice the technique from start to finish, twice a day. Do this for about a week.

At the end of the week, assess your progress. Do you feel comfortable with your images? Do you feel you can control them? If you do not find your images accurate or totally believable, you may need to adjust them—or find entirely new images. Go back to Chapter 7 and review the properties of subjective and objective imagery. Look at the pain-interpretation charts. Keep searching until you find the right images. You must decide for yourself what they will be, but you will know them when you find them. Like finding a pair of trousers that fit just right, you will be able to sense when you have found the images that fit you.

Most important of all, don't get discouraged. This

is no different from learning any other skill. You stumbled and fell repeatedly before you learned to walk. Olympic skaters spend a lot of time on the seat of their pants before they master the moves that make them champions.

We have suggested that you begin by practicing in a relatively pain-free environment, but don't be afraid to try imagery when an actual episode of pain strikes. Concentrate on completely controlling your image. Stay relaxed and allow your imagery to work. Don't let yourself back away from the pain—let your image confront it. Use your successes, and your failures, to perfect your imaging. Again, you might find it helpful to track your efforts by using the pain-control scale in Chapter 1.

How long will it take to feel some real reduction in pain? Some people find immediate results. For most people, however, it takes two to three weeks to become comfortable enough with their images to start controlling their pain. And it often takes more than a month to master the technique.

There is one more thing to keep in mind. In fact, it's something to look forward to. As a by-product of mastering the guided pain-control protocol, you will find that you no longer need to go through all the steps we have outlined here. The whole process will become automatic. Like the boy we told you about who just had to say "Hands, you're hot," or the woman who just had to think of a metal bar to call up the imaginal response that relieved her headaches, you will find that the process becomes automatic for you too. The entire imaging process, through practice and repetition, will become integrated into an almost instantaneous autogenic experience. You will have trained your body and mind to respond to your prompt. A single invocation of the prompt will trigger relaxation and communication between your mind and body. It will all happen instinctively, bringing you relief from your pain. Finally.

SIDEBAR—A SAFE HAVEN

Sad to say, there are some instances when pain-control imagery doesn't seem to work. A few of our patients have been unable to create an effective prompt for their pain because they haven't been able to develop any clear image of the pain. Either they're in such terrible pain that they can't effectively describe it, or they're having trouble understanding what prompt could possibly counteract the pain.

For them, there is still one imagery technique that works. And it can work for you too. If all else fails, you can remove yourself from the world of pain by creating a sanctuary—a safe haven—where pain is not allowed.

This technique is actually a form of subjective imagery. You create a subjective image that counteracts the pain by taking you away from the objective world.

Search your experiences, your memories, or your

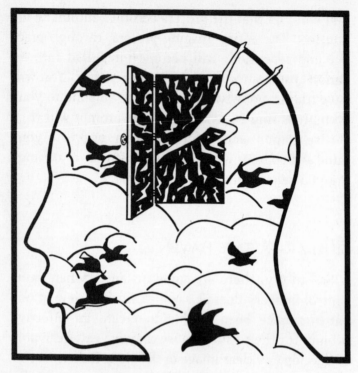

A Safe Haven

fantasies for a safe, peaceful, comfortable place—a place you can go to whenever your pain becomes too much to bear.

Your haven may be your favorite room, or a bed, a beach, a car driving on the open highway through the desert flowers; or it could be a more exotic sanctuary—another planet or a cloud, any place where you can feel protected and serene.

Prepare your haven in advance; have it ready before your pain comes. Invoke all your senses to experience it. Feel what the place is like. Smell the fresh grass, or the sea air, or the smoke from the fireplace. Hear its sounds and feel its textures—your softest most comfortable clothes, the ground or floor underfoot. See your sanctuary completely, in clear, comprehensive detail. Taste whatever there is to taste. Know it completely.

Explore the place that you've created, this special place where there is no pain. Don't dream of this place as you might wish upon a star, with no real hope of your wish coming true. Go to your sanctuary body and soul, with all your senses active and probing. If you create this haven halfheartedly, your mind won't accept it.

Begin by using your relaxation regimen. Find a quiet place where you won't be disturbed. Breathe deeply, using belly breathing; detach yourself from the weight of your body; call upon your calming image to relax your body and mind.

Now go to your safe haven.

Image a door that leads to your safe haven. Step through the door. Close the door. Leave behind the outside world—and your pain. In effect, you are using your imagery to cut yourself off from the rest of the world. The image you create of your haven is your way of isolating yourself from all outside stimuli. By doing so, you can keep pain at bay. Stay in your safe haven until the pain subsides, or until you are comfortable enough to open the door and rejoin the rest of the world.

PUTTING IT ALL TOGETHER

Here is a summary of the steps for using each type of imagery.

Subjective Imagery
A. Finding your autogenic prompt
    1. Determine what your pain feels like.
    2. Create a vivid image of your pain.
    3. Find a prompt you can use to counteract your pain.
B. Using pain-control imagery
    1. Begin with your relaxation regimen.
        a. Start a slow, regular rhythm of belly breathing.
        b. Detach your mind from the weight of your body.
        c. Use calming imagery to relax your body and mind.
    2. Concentrate on your image of your pain.
    3. Concentrate on your prompt to counteract the pain.
    4. Image your prompt relieving the pain.
Practice the protocol until pain control becomes an autogenic response.

Objective Imagery
A. Finding your autogenic prompt
    1. Investigate what causes your pain.

2. Create a vivid image of the physical cause of your pain.

3. Find a prompt you can use to counteract the cause of your pain.

B. Using pain-control imagery

   1. Begin with your relaxation regimen.

      a. Start a slow, regular rhythm of belly breathing.

      b. Detach your mind from the weight of your body.

      c. Use calming imagery to relax your body and mind.

   2. Concentrate on your image of the cause of your pain.

   3. Concentrate on your prompt to counteract the pain.

   4. Image your prompt relieving the pain.

Practice the protocol until pain control becomes an autogenic response.

Safe Haven

A. Creating a safe haven

   1. Think of a place—real or fantasy—where you would like to go in order to escape your pain.

   2. Create a vivid, detailed image of your safe haven. Include sights, sounds, textures, etc.

B. Going there

   1. Begin with your relaxation regimen.

      a. Start a slow, regular rhythm of belly breathing.

   b. Detach your mind from the weight of your
       body.
   c. Use calming imagery to relax your body
       and mind.
2. Concentrate on your image of your safe haven.
3. Image yourself entering your safe haven, leaving your pain behind.

CHAPTER 10

Other Vantage Points

Your pain is unique, yours alone. But others hurt as much as you do, and you can gain valuable insights from their experiences.

The case histories that follow will enable you to see the imagery protocol in action, and, we hope, provide the guidance and inspiration you'll need to make the process a useful element of your own personal pain-control regimen.

GWEN

Gwen, who is thirty-four, hurt her upper back and neck in a car accident about two years ago. Since the accident, Gwen has suffered frequent episodes of extremely uncomfortable pain and frightening numbness. When it comes, the pain is so severe that it is almost impossible for her to walk or even stand. She can find some slight relief only by sitting in a firm chair or by lying down.

Gwen is a banquet director. Her job requires her to meet with clients and to attend many social functions. Gwen's duties force her into almost constant motion, and she's expected to be pleasant and enthusiastic.

Neurologists, orthopedic surgeons, chiropractors, and acupuncturists have all treated Gwen at one time or another, but none of the doctors or therapists could identify the specific cause of Gwen's pain. When Gwen sued the person responsible for her car accident, a diagnostic test called thermography was used to determine if Gwen's pain could be detected and measured. Thermography is a diagnostic procedure that scans the body for temperature variations in suspected pain sites.

Gwen's thermographic scan proved inconclusive; so she lost her case. No pain, the courts said. The decision added depression and rage to Gwen's collection of frustrations.

Did the thermography results mean that Gwen wasn't in pain, that she was making it all up? Of course not. The experience of pain, as we've said before, can't be measured, pictured, or truly understood by anyone except the person experiencing it.

Gwen was desperate by the time she came to us. We asked her to describe her pain. "I have the most severe attacks about two or three times a week," she said. "It feels like a knife is cutting from the middle of my back, right through my shoulder blades, and up to the left side of my neck. Then, after the hot, searing pain subsides, I go numb. It's sort of a sickly numbness, a tingling, almost the way you feel when you have your hand underneath your head and you sleep on it all night. A cold, dead feeling."

We told Gwen that she was describing her pain in too many different ways and that she needed to isolate a central focus for her painful sensations.

"I would say that the cold numbness is the feeling that makes me most uncomfortable," Gwen decided, after some thought. "I can't turn my head to the left when the numbness comes because it hurts so much. When the attacks start, I almost feel as if I want to have someone slap me on the back, and sometimes I've even asked people to do that, to get the blood pumping there, to get some feeling back in that area."

We asked Gwen what happens when people actually slap the area of her back where the pain seems to originate.

"Well, sometimes it makes me feel as if I am going to get the blood circulating again, and it feels somewhat better," Gwen said. "But most of the time, it's so deeply numb in that area, it almost makes me nauseous when my skin is touched or massaged in any way during an attack."

After lengthy discussion, we suggested to Gwen that perhaps an image of heat would be effective in counteracting the cold dead numbness that she continued to identify as the dominant element of her pain experience.

We taught Gwen the imagery protocol and encouraged her to practice. Within three weeks she reported back to us.

"This is going to sound funny," Gwen said. "I experimented with all kinds of heat images. The one that seemed to work best was when I imaged myself naked, standing in a large cylindrical tub of warm water—not too hot. The warm water was circulating around me in kind of a slow whirlpool, relaxing my back and neck muscles, and allowing more blood to flow to the numb areas. It really helped.

"The funny part is that I felt very uncomfortable imaging myself naked when I was at work with other people. So, for work I imaged a warm water bottle tied around my back, right over the spot where the numbness is at its worst. The effect was about the same."

Gwen was not, at this point, in complete control of her pain. She had just begun to practice imagery, after all. But she was off to a fine start, and she progressed nicely. Now her pain doesn't interfere so seriously with her career or her life. She has told us that with every passing week, she feels herself strengthening her imagery skills and becoming more optimistic about her future.

No one rattled any caribou bones over Gwen's back, or sprinkled her with magic dust. Imagery is not voodoo, or hocus-pocus, or a parlor trick done with mirrors and blue smoke. Imagery is a natural ability, a mental skill that can be developed in the same way that physical skills or public-speaking skills or musical skills can be developed. You don't have to believe in a swami or an ancient deity to make imagery work. It's a very real, deeply expressive language of the mind.

TAMARA

Tamara is a forty-one-year-old housewife who came to us for help in coping with severe migraine headaches. It was obvious that Tamara had once been an extremely attractive woman. When we first met her, however, years of pain had drawn and hardened her features and drained her spirit. She was deeply depressed, primarily because of her inability to manage her chronic pain.

Tamara is responsible for taking care of a large home and five children. Most of her energy goes into cooking, cleaning, laundry, maintaining the household budget, and coordinating her children's many after-school activities. By the time we met her, Tamara's headaches had become so devastating that they had made a shambles of her everyday life. She had become short-tempered, somewhat distant, and unresponsive sexually. She became reclusive, leaving her house only when absolutely necessary.

When Tamara's headaches came, they stayed for as long as a day and a half, bringing with them nausea and what Tamara described as a "sense of doom"—a feeling that her life was going to end.

Between migraine attacks, Tamara lived like a zombie. She felt overwhelmed, lonely, and utterly helpless. She didn't see any hope for a better future; so she waited, walking the hallways of her home aimlessly, dreading the time when her next attack would descend upon her. She was depressed, like many chronic pain sufferers, because she couldn't see any hope that she would ever feel better.

Our first interview with Tamara revealed that her headaches had begun shortly after the birth of her first child. She said that she had been experiencing tremendous migraine pain about three times a week ever since.

Surprisingly, Tamara had sought little medical treatment before we met her. We sent her to her doctor for a full neurological examination, but Tamara's neurological tests turned up no cause for her headaches. Nevertheless, the drug Cafergot, which constricts blood vessels, was prescribed, and the drug reduced Tamara's pain slightly. But it was not effective enough to provide any significant relief.

Eventually, the fear of pain had become as powerful as the pain itself. "I live in constant fear of the pain coming," she said. "I never know when it will strike next and that keeps me from ever relaxing or having a halfway decent time."

Tamara felt trapped, and, at one low point, she wondered if death might be better than her pain. "There are times when I fantasize about taking a loaded gun and putting it to my head and pulling the trigger, just to relieve the tension," Tamara said. "Well, I don't really want to kill myself, but I have to admit, I often wish I could get rid of this pain in one fell swoop."

Tamara's pain was a powerful presence, a demanding entity that pushed aside the rest of her life.

"When I get an attack," she told us, "I don't care about anybody but myself. I don't care about the kids' problems, or my husband's. I can't do anything. I curl up in a ball under the covers and try to ride out the storm."

This recollection brought tears to Tamara's eyes. After she regained her composure she told us what she wished for: "I wish someone would rescue me from this pain. I don't know who. Is there a pill, or, maybe some machine? Isn't there something we can do to stop this pain right now? I can't take it anymore."

But what couldn't she take anymore? What was her pain like? We asked Tamara to describe how her pain made her feel, and we were pleasantly surprised when she offered a quick and specific response.

"I feel a sense of dread sweeping through my body," she said. "Then, within a half-hour or so, the pain begins at my left temple and runs down the back of my head, around my ear. It pulsates at first, like too much blood being pumped into my head too quickly. Then, as time goes on—and these things last a long, long time—it feels as if somebody is pounding a big bass drum, the kind you see in symphony orchestras. The pounding gets louder and louder and louder, and it's all inside my head, next to my ear. It feels as if my head is going to explode. Sometimes I bury my head under pillows and put as much pressure on them as I can, with my hands pushing down on the pillows. I try to smother the pain, but it doesn't work. That drum inside my head keeps beating."

Since an image as direct and clear as a bass drum could be managed, we realized that if Tamara could create an image to counteract the drum, then perhaps her pain could be alleviated. Any image of the drum being muffled or rendered unplayable could help her. We told Tamara this, and explained how imagery works (much as we've explained it to you). She understood the nuances of the imagery protocol quickly and seemed eager to try the procedure.

Some weeks later, Tamara returned to report a measure of success. She had used the imagery technique several times, and she felt that she was managing her pain much better, although she wasn't able to make it disappear completely.

"Whenever the drum starts beating," Tamara said, "I image a thick layer of soft cotton being draped over the drum. When the mallet beats against the drum, the soft material absorbs the impact and muffles the sound." To test the strength of her image, Tamara goes a step further. "I image doing all I can to make a sound on that big bass drum with its soft cotton cover, and when I can't make any noise that alone seems to make me feel better. It keeps the pulsing feeling from being so strong and so painful.'' The more Tamara could feel the silence of the muffled drum, the less pain she experienced.

Tamara is doing very well now, we're happy to say. She says that her life is much more pleasurable, and she smiles more often every time we see her. Encouraged by her newly discovered ability to somewhat control her chronic pain, Tamara has taken a more aggressive role in her medical treatment. She and her doctors have worked out a safe, effective medication schedule. Tamara's rapidly expanding imagery skills, combined with the prescription analgesics, have resulted in fewer and far less powerful headaches for Tamara. On the pain-control scale we introduced in Chapter 1, Tamara has dialed down her pain from 10 to less than zero.

Tamara and Gwen both were quick to tell us exactly how their pain felt. Their own heavily symbolic, highly personalized descriptions of pain pointed quickly to effective therapeutic prompts. Harold had to travel quite a different path.

HAROLD

Harold is a professor of industrial psychology at a major midwestern university. Although he had suffered for years with chronic migraine headaches,

Harold didn't come to us for help in managing his pain. Professional curiosity prompted his initial visit. Harold had read of our work with pain-control imagery and wanted to discuss the results of our research.

It wasn't until after we outlined our clinical protocol that Harold revealed his own problems with chronic pain. When we offered to teach him the protocol, he at first declined.

"I really don't see how imagery can help," he said.

We asked Harold to humor us, and he agreed to try the protocol—more as a theoretical experiment than as a practical self-treatment.

Harold described his headaches in precise, accurate medical terms. He had read a great deal about migraine headaches and had even contacted the National Headache Foundation in Illinois for its most current literature. Harold was very clear about what was happening inside his head. His migraine pain was of the vascular variety, he said, and he knew exactly what that meant.

This is how Harold described his pain: "I'm quite familiar with vascular headaches and arterial dilation and I know that only arterial constrictors will reduce the pain. For some reason, though, I haven't been very successful with the medications I've been taking."

We told Harold that understanding the source of his pain wasn't enough. We wanted Harold to talk about his experience of pain—how it made him feel, not where it came from.

"I don't know if you saw it," Harold said, "but recently on TV there was a movie about Abraham Lincoln and his wife Mary Todd, who had tremendously painful migraines on a fairly regular basis. I remember watching the show, because I'm a Civil War buff anyway, and there was a scene in which Mary Tyler Moore, who played Lincoln's wife, began to whine and cry that she was about to get one of her headaches. She had a look of utter terror on her face.

"Well, I identified with that scene," Harold said. "When my headaches start, I really feel as if I'm going to panic. I wish I could run away from them somehow. I wish there was a way to avoid them, just as I would avoid a punch thrown at me. When you see a punch coming, you duck, or you block it. But even though my headaches are somewhat telegraphed, there isn't anything I can do."

We suggested to Harold that the pain-control protocol might be something he could do. Harold replied that, while he found imagery interesting from a psychological perspective, he doubted its value as a therapeutic process. "I really can't see how I can somehow wish my pain away," he said. "I'm fairly intelligent, and if all I needed to do was to wish my pain away, I would have done it long ago."

We assured Harold that imagery had nothing to do with wishing or with intelligence; that it was simply the mind's most accessible link with the body. We reminded Harold of our own successes with clinical imagery, and we showed him evidence compiled by other doctors of imagery's effectiveness.

"Don't get me wrong," Harold said. "I want desperately to believe in this, and I'll give it a try. I haven't gotten through a book in months. I've been sleeping poorly and I've fallen behind in getting my curriculum in order. My job could be in danger unless I do something about dealing with these headaches."

We told Harold that he didn't have to "believe" in anything, that imagery required no special faith, that it was not a mystical experience. "Keep an open mind and be willing to try," we said to Harold. "That's all we ask."

We again attempted to draw out Harold's sensory impressions of his chronic pain. "Well, I know my headaches are due to vascular dilation," Harold said. "When they occur I feel this tremendous pressure right at the front and near the top of my head. It's almost as if the blood is just pouring in. I usually get nauseous when the attacks come. When the headaches finally subside, I feel such utter relief, such indescribable pleasure I wish I could package the feeling and take it as a pill to combat the pain from the headaches the rest of the time."

It seemed clear that, given Harold's personality, and his comprehensive knowledge of the physical aspects of his migraines, the objective-imagery protocol offered the best chance for success. Harold had a clear and detailed objective understanding of the mechanics of his pain. We felt he could draw on that understanding to find an image that would respond to the pain.

Harold underwent imagery training, and soon afterward, he came to see us again with a very interesting story.

"I had an awful attack a couple of days after seeing you guys, and the imagery technique didn't work for me at all. In fact," Harold said, "I didn't spend much time trying to use it. The pain was so horrible, I lost all sense of hope and all knowledge of what I was supposed to do to help myself.

"But then, just yesterday, I burned my hand on the stove. It hurt like a sonofabitch, and there was no ice in the freezer and no burn cream in the medicine cabinet. My hand started to blister and the throbbing was terrible. I decided, what the hell, I'll give it a try. I imaged that I had ice on my hand, and that I was freezing the area I'd burned. I totally ad-libbed this. I had no warning that this burn was coming but just imaging the ice seemed to help tremendously. I was impressed."

We were impressed too. We congratulated Harold on his impromptu success and naturally encouraged him to practice the imagery protocol to manage his headaches. Harold promised to do so, and when we saw him two weeks later, he reported resounding success: "I've been using clips to clamp down on my arteries whenever the headache starts," Harold said. "I know the clips will slow down the blood rushing into my head.

"It really works! Imaging a control of the blood flow is making it happen, or, at least, it's making me feel like it happens. I don't care, I feel much better."

Harold now recommends our pain-control system in his job as an industrial psychologist, and he teaches imagery techniques to medical directors of the corporations that employ him as a consultant. Harold tells his clients that imagery techniques can be a valuable tool in rehabilitating employees suffering from chronic pain. He speaks from the best personal experience.

Harold's problem was that, although he knew very well how and why he was hurting, he didn't really know what his pain felt like. George had an entirely different problem. George could not understand his pain at all, and neither could his doctors. For him, an "escape" image was needed.

GEORGE

George had been a mail carrier for eighteen years, and he had never had a bad day. He was a strong, healthy, robust man. He'd never even been to a doctor.

About two years ago, George felt his first physical

agony—back pain that became so severe that he was forced to give up his mail route for a hospital bed and traction. Doctors were confused. They could find no medical reason for George's pain.

After much discussion, the doctors theorized that George's pain was simply the result of his body breaking down after almost two decades of hard work. After all, they reasoned, George's route was several miles long, and he walked it every day.

George missed a lot of work, and eventually Workmen's Compensation insisted that he undertake a rehabilitation program known as "work hardening." Every day, George went to a therapy facility and practiced activities similar to those required in his job. George would bend down to pick up sacks of mail. He would sling the bags over his shoulders and walk several miles along the facilities track. His back pain subsided only slightly, however, so he was sent to see us.

We asked George to describe the experience of his pain. He couldn't. "I really don't know," George said. "I have no idea how to explain it. All I know is it hurts. It's sort of pinching, sort of hot, just a whole lot of pain. I have a hell of a time walking for more than a block before I have to sit down, or stand against a tree, just for the firmness of the trunk."

George was bewildered by his pain. "I can't do the things I used to do," he said. "I don't know what's happening to me. My doctors don't either. All I know is I've spent a lot of money and I've lost a lot of time on the job and things are pretty bad at home, and I've got to figure out a way to get out of this thing."

We asked George to go home for a couple of days and spend the time in careful concentration. We needed a specific description of his pain to help him control it.

When George returned things weren't any better. "I tried to isolate some major sensation," he said. "But I really can't get any specific handle on it. It just hurts a lot. I did notice that I break into a cold sweat sometimes when the pain is really bad, but that's about all I can tell you."

Because George seemed to have absolutely no sensory image of his pain, either subjective or objective, we suggested that he try to recall his least painful body position. This was a concept that George could handle.

"The most comfortable position for me is lying on an extra firm mattress or sitting in a good stiff chair," he said. "That seems to be the only thing I can do to reduce my pain. The painkillers I've been taking help a little, but I still can't walk for more than a block, no matter what I take."

We suggested to George that he adapt the pain-control protocol, and use a customized version of the imagery technique. We told him to image himself in the comfortable positions he described—lying down on a firm mattress or sitting in a stiff chair, whatever helped him with his pain.

A week later, George came to see us again. He was

quietly optimistic. "It really is amazing how effective simple things can be," George told us. "I tried walking around the neighborhood high-school track, a quarter-mile. When I started feeling pain, I experimented with doing exactly what you told me to do. I felt myself sitting in a strong hard-backed chair, and I was able to keep walking. The pain didn't go away or anything," he said, "but I was able to tolerate it."

George seems to be progressing toward complete control of his chronic pain. His improvement is slow but consistent; he feels a little better each time we see him. He is back to work part-time and he's hopeful about his future. George's case is a clear example of a common problem: the inability to articulate—in any terms—the sensation of chronic pain. An effective therapeutic image cannot be created when there is no definite sensory impression to counteract.

Because George could not confront his pain, he used imagery to escape it. If you're having similar difficulties in defining your pain in sensory terms, try an escape image in place of a control prompt. Take yourself away from your pain to a safe, quiet sanctuary. As George's experience illustrates, your escape image need not be elaborate. Use the escape technique whenever you're distracted by your pain, or when you're simply exhausted and a control image is difficult to summon. Take a vacation from your pain.

George was able to escape his pain without isolating himself from the rest of the world. For some pain sufferers, however, a more complete escape is needed, an escape to a safe haven. As the following case history shows, it is possible to escape to a safe haven even under the most trying circumstances.

JOAN

Joan is a charming wife and mother in her mid-thirties confronting one of the most frightening of life's nightmares—cancer. A few years ago, she noticed a small lump on one of her breasts, but she kept putting off going to the doctor to have it examined. When she finally did, the doctor discovered a malignant tumor. A section of the breast was removed, but a few months later the doctor discovered more cancer. A full mastectomy had to be performed.

Joan seemed to make a full recovery after that. However, fourteen months later she started complaining of back pain. She returned to the doctor, who confirmed her worst fear. The cancer had returned, and it was spreading throughout her body. Joan now faced a barrage of debilitating radiation and chemotherapy treatments.

Joan suffered the consequences common to those undergoing radical cancer treatments. The radiation treatments caused her hair to fall out. The chemotherapy was worse, ravaging her system with nausea and pain. "It's like swallowing Drano and then waiting for the onslaught," she told us. "It's twenty-four hours of hell."

Joan came to us searching for a way to deal with the agony of the chemotherapy. In our discussions with her, it became clear that the intensity of her pain and the range of factors causing it made an escape image the only viable alternative. We explained the safe haven imagery to her and suggested she try to think of a sanctuary she would like to escape to. Joan considered our suggestions and also thought about her very uncertain future. She came up with an image that might seem odd and ironic, but for her it has proven to be quite effective. The safe haven she has imaged is heaven.

The image came to her as she fantasized about exploring the unknown. She found it comforting to develop a picture of what might lie ahead. She was able to create a vivid, detailed image of her safe haven.

To go to her safe haven, she closes her eyes and feels her spirit leave her body. It travels down a long hallway on a transport made of a beam of light. Along the way, she sees the dead friends and relatives with whom she might be reunited, as well as famous celebrities and historical leaders she will now get to meet.

At the end of the hallway, she enters a room made of soft, white walls, moist and fluffy like clouds. Her favorite music is playing. Anything she wants appears to her. A soft, soothing voice tells her, "You're safe, you're home; nothing can hurt you." She lies on a soft bed and feels a plush, fluffy blanket cover her. In her haven, Joan feels safe and warm.

Joan's safe haven has helped her escape the ravages of chemotherapy; it's her mental equivalent of biting the bullet. Going to her safe haven doesn't eliminate the pain, but it gives her something to focus on that makes the pain more bearable. Finding her safe haven has helped her keep her spirits up as she continues her daunting battle with cancer.

Joan's experience is obviously an extreme case, but it demonstrates once again the power of imagery. If you cannot conquer your pain, you can at least use imagery to escape from it and keep it at bay.

A FINAL GLANCE

We hope we've helped you see and understand that a pain-free future is possible. We realize that it won't be easy.

Accept that fact. Commit to it. Be active and aggressive in accepting and managing your chronic pain. Believe us when we tell you the results will be worth the work and concentration required.

Practice pain-control imagery until you've mastered every nuance. Make it a natural element of your mental processes. Our patients have been able to use imagery to hurt less, and so can you.

You can overcome your pain. There's no trickery involved, no sorcery, no deception. The power rests with you, in your own mind. You can image yourself free of pain.

APPENDIX

Support Groups and Other Organizations

You are not alone in your search for relief from pain. We supply in this section many of the organizations and support groups you can turn to for information and advice.

In particular, we invite you to contact us at the International Society for Imagery Science (ISIS). We are a nonprofit organization headed by a board of directors drawn from the psychological, neuropsychological, and medical communities. We are a forum for researchers, we conduct our own research, and we serve as a repository for the collection of studies and reports on the application of imagery to pain control. We offer support groups and referrals to doctors who specialize in pain control. You can get in touch with us at the following address:

1750 East Golf Road, Suite 324
Schaumburg, IL 60173
Phone: (312) 240-4040
Ken Dachman, Chairman
John Lyons, Executive Director

Other groups, arranged in alphabetical order, are listed below.

American Council for Healthful Living
439 Main Street
Orange, NJ 07050
Phone: (201) 674-7476
Raymond Siegener, Executive Director

American Council on Science and Health
1995 Broadway, 18th Floor
New York, NY 10023
Phone: (212) 362-7044
Elizabeth M. Whelen, Executive Director

American Foundation for Alternative Health Care, Research and Development (AFAHCRD)
25 Landfield Avenue
Monticello, NY 12701
Phone: (914) 794-8181
Edwin M. Field, Executive Director

American Healing Association (AHA)
c/o Rev. Brian Zink
Glendale, CA 91206
Rev. Brian Zink, Executive Officer

American Health Care Advisory Association (AHCAA)
1825 I Street, N.W., Suite 400
Washington, DC 20006
Donovan F. Ward, M.D., Director

American Healthcare Institute
1919 Pennsylvania Avenue, N.W., Suite 703
Washington, DC 20006
Phone: (202) 293-2840
Merlin K. Du Val, M.D., President

American Health Foundation
320 East 43d Street
New York, NY 10017
Phone: (212) 953-1900
Ernst L. Wynder, M.D., President

American Imagery Association (AIA)
4016 Third Avenue
San Diego, CA 92103
Phone: (619) 298-7502
Dennis J. Gersten, M.D., President

American International Reiki Association
2210 Wilshire Boulevard, Suite 831
Santa Monica, CA 90403
Phone: (213) 394-6220
Yesnie Carrington, Director

American Juvenile Arthritis Organization
1314 Spring Street
Atlanta, GA 30309
Phone: (404) 872-7100
Linda Wetherbee, Contact

American Pain Society (APS)
1615 L Street, N.W., Suite 925
Washington, DC 20036
Phone: (202) 296-9200
Marie W. Klemann, Executive Director

American Rheumatism Association
17 Executive Park Drive, N.E., Suite 480
Atlanta, GA 30329
Phone: (404) 633-3777
Mark Andrejeski, Executive Vice President

Archaeus Project
2402 University Avenue
St. Paul, MN 55114
Phone: (612) 641-0177
Dennis Stillings, Director

Arthritis Care
6 Grosvenor Crescent
London SW1X 7ER, England
Phone: 1 2350902
P. Turner, Contact

Arthritis Foundation
1314 Spring Street, N.W.
Atlanta, GA 30309
Phone: (404) 872-7100
Clifford M. Clarke, CAE, President

Association for People with Arthritis
P.O. Box 954
Six Commercial Street
Hicksville, NY 11802

European League Against Rheumatism
(Ligue Européenne contre le Rhumatisme)
Promenadengasse 18
CH-8001 Zurich, Switzerland
Phone: 1 2524866
Fred K. Wyss, Executive Secretary

Foundation for Health
337 East Avenue
Watertown, NY
Phone: (315) 782-6664
George Bonadino, Executive Director

Gerson Institute
P.O. Box 430
Bonita, CA 92002
Phone: (619) 267-1150
Charlotte Gerson, President

Holistic Health Havens
3419 Thom Boulevard
Las Vegas, NV 89106
Phone: (702) 645-1799
Dr. Joseph M. Kadans, President

International Association for the Study of Pain (IASP)
909 N.E. 43d Street, Suite 306
Seattle, WA
Phone: (206) 547-6409
Louisa E. Jones, Executive Officer

International Imagery Association (IIA)
P.O. Box 1046
Bronx, NY 10471
Akhter Ahsen, Chairman

International League Against Rheumatism
c/o Charles M. Plotz, M.D.
SUNY Downstate Medical Center
450 Clarkson Avenue
Brooklyn, NY 11203
Phone: (718) 270-2422
Charles M. Plotz, M.D., Treasurer

International Society for Mental Imagery Techniques in
Psychotherapy and Psychology
(Société Internationale des Techniques d'Imagerie
Mentale—SITIM)
6, rue des Ursulines
F-75005 Paris, France
Phone: 1 43269892
Dr. André Virel, President

National Chronic Pain Outreach Association (NCPO)
4922 Hampden Lane
Bethesda, MD 20814
Phone: (301) 652-4948
Laura S. Hitchcock, Ph.D., President

National Committee on the Treatment of Intractable Pain
(NCTIP)
P.O. Box 9553, Friendship Station
Washington, DC 20016
Phone: (202) 944-8140
Judith H. Quattlebaum, President

National Headache Foundation
5252 North Western Avenue
Chicago, IL 60625
Phone: (312) 878-5558
Seymour Diamond, M.D., Executive Director

National Head Injury Foundation
333 Turnpike Road
Southborough, MA 01772
Phone: (617) 485-9950
Marilyn Price Spivack, President

National Health Federation (NHF)
P.O. Box 688
Monrovia, CA 91016
Phone: (818) 357-2181
Maureen Salaman, President

National Reye's Syndrome Foundation
426 North Lewis
Bryan, OH 43506
Phone: (419) 636-2679
John E. Freudenberger, President

Natural Marketing Association
22704 Ventura Boulevard, Suite 506
Woodland Hills, CA 91364
Phone: (808) 702-0888
Steve Gorman, President

ODPHP National Health Information Center
P.O. Box 1133
Washington, DC 20013
Phone: (301) 565-4167
Linda Malcolm, Project Director

Pan American League Against Rheumatism
c/o Dr. Hugo E. Jasin
Department of Internal Medicine
University of Texas Health Care Center
5323 Harry Hines Boulevard
Dallas, TX 75235
Phone: (214) 688-3466
Dr. Hugo E. Jasin, Treasurer

Roger Wyburn-Mason and Jack M. Blount Foundation
for the Eradication of Rheumatoid Disease
Route 4, Box 137
Franklin, TN 37064
Phone: (615) 646-1030
Perry A. Chapdelaine, Executive Director

Touch for Health Foundation
1174 North Lake Avenue
Pasadena, CA 91104
Phone: (818) 794-1181
W. W. Scott Rubel, Administrative Assistant

A Wellness Center, Inc.
15 East 40th Street, Suite 704
New York, NY 10016
Phone: (212) 532-4286
Dr. Hugo W. Roberts, Director

Suggested Reading

Achterberg, Jeanne. *Imagery In Healing: Shamanism and Modern Medicine*. Boston: New Science Library, 1985.

Arthritis Foundation. *Arthritis: The Basic Facts*. Atlanta, GA: Arthritis Foundation, 1976.

Beecher, H. K. "Pain in Men Wounded in Battle." *Annals of Surgery*, 1946.

Bennett, Hal, and Mike Samuels. *The Well Body Book*. New York: Random House, 1973.

Benson, Herbert. *The Mind/Body Effect*. New York: Simon & Schuster, 1983.

Benson, Herbert, and Miriam Z. Klipper. *The Relaxation Response*. New York: Avon, 1976.

Borysenko, Joan. *Minding the Body, Mending the Mind*. Reading, MA: Addison-Wesley, 1987.

Bresler, David E., and Richard Trubo. *Free Yourself from Pain*. New York: Simon & Schuster, 1979.

Bright, Deborah. *Creative Relaxation*. New York: Harcourt Brace Jovanovich, 1979.

Cousins, Norman. *Anatomy of an Illness as Perceived by the Patient*. New York: Bantam, 1981.

Faraday, Ann. *Dream Power*. New York: Berkley, 1973.

Garfield, Patricia. *Creative Dreaming*. New York: Simon & Schuster, 1974.

Gawain, Shakti. *Creative Visualization*. New York: Bantam, 1979.

Gillespie, Peggy, and Lynn Bechtel. *Less Stress in Thirty Days*. New York: New American Library, 1986.

Hendler, N., and J. A. Fenton. *Coping With Chronic Pain*. New York: Clarkson N. Potter, 1979.

Hittleman, Richard. *Yoga: Twenty-Eight Day Exercise Plan*. New York: Bantam, 1973.

Kurland, Howard D. *Back Pain: Quick Relief Without Drugs*. New York: Simon & Schuster, 1981.

Leshan, Lawrence. *How to Meditate*. New York: Bantam, 1984.

Locke, Steven, and Douglas Colligan. *The Healer Within: The New Medicine of Mind and Body*. New York: E. P. Dutton, 1986.

Luthe, W., ed. *Autogenic Therapy*. New York: Grune & Stratton, 1969.

Melzack, R. *The Puzzle of Pain*. New York: Basic Books, 1973.

Morse, Donald R. *Stress for Success*. New York: Van Nostrand Reinhold, 1979.

Olshan, N. H. *Power over Your Pain Without Drugs*. New York: Beanfort Books, 1983.

Oyle, Irving. *The Healing Mind*. New York: Pocket Books, 1975.

Pelletier, Kenneth R. *Mind as Healer, Mind as Slayer*. New York: Delacorte, 1977.

Richardson, A. *Mental Imagery*. New York: Springer, 1969.

Samuels, Mike, and Nancy Samuels. *Seeing With the Mind's Eye*. New York: Random House, 1975.

Shaw, Eva. *Sixty Second Shiatsu: How to Energize, Erase Pain & Conquer Tension in One Minute*. Bedford, MA: Mills & Sanderson, 1987.

Shealy, C. Norman. *The Pain Game*. Berkeley: Celestial Arts, 1976.

Siegel, Bernie S. *Peace, Love and Healing*. New York: Harper & Row, 1989.

————. *Love, Medicine and Miracles*. New York: Harper & Row, 1986.

Simonton, O., S. M. Simonton, and James Creighton. *Getting Well Again*. New York: Bantam, 1980.

Index

Acute pain, functions of, 8
Agrippa, Marcus Vipsanius, 25
Ali, Muhammad, 28
American Council for Healthful Living, 146
American Council on Science and Health, 146
American Foundation for Alternative Health Care, Research and Development (AFAHCRD), 146
American Healing Association (AHA), 146
American Health Care Advisory Association (AHCAA), 146
American Healthcare Institute, 146
American Health Foundation, 147
American Imagery Association (AIA), 147
American International Reiki Association, 147
American Juvenile Arthritis Organization, 147
American Pain Society (APS), 147
American Rheumatism Association, 148
Angina, 96–97
Anxiety, 106
Archaeus Project, 148
Arthritis, 99–101
Arthritis Care, 148
Arthritis Foundation, 148
Association for People with Arthritis, 148

Athletic training technique, 44–46
Autogenic prompt, 87–89, 102, 115, 116–17
    definition of, 87–88
    objective imagery and, 98, 99–101
    subjective imagery and, 92, 93, 95–97
Autonomic nervous system, 31, 36–37

Back pain, 17–18, 100, 125–28, 139–42
Barban, Lisa, 29
Beecher, H. K., 26
Biofeedback, 47
Bitterness, 23–24
Blaming, avoidance of, 23
Blindness, imagery and, 40–41
Breathing, effective, 107–9, 116
Bresler, David E., 51–52

Cancer, 52, 100, 142–44
Cerebral cortex, 31
Children, imagery skills of, 56
Chronic pain. See Pain, chronic
Clinical imagery (guided imagery).
    See also Pain-control imagery
    definition of, 51
Color, exercises for, 71–74
Concentration, 57, 74–78, 106–7
Conrad, Joseph, 39
Craig, Vernon, 28
Creativity, 81–83

Daily life, assessment of impact of pain on, 19–22
DCS (dorsal column stimulator), 15
Death, drugs and, 12
Depression, victim mentality and, 23–24
Depth, 71–74
Despair, 23–24
Detachment, relaxation and, 109–12
Details, 58, 74–79
Dorsal Column Stimulator (DCS), 15
Douglas, Bobby, 28
Drugs, pain-control, 11–13

Economic costs of pain, 7, 11
Effective imagery exercises, 64–86
    for color, depth, and spatial integration, 71–74
    for concentration and attention to detail, 74–78
    creativity, 81–83
    for feelings about details, 78–79
    hearing, 69–70
    for memory, 79–81
    scale for, 65–67, 70, 71
    touch, 68–69
    vision, 67–68
    for vivid, extended image, 83–85
Electrical stimulation, 11, 14–15
Endorphins, 31
Epinephrine, 32
European League Against Rheumatism, 149
Exercises, 57–86, 103
    breathing, 108–9
    effective imagery. *See* Effective imagery exercises
    relaxation and, 108–12
    sensory deprivation, 59–64
        hearing, 61–62
        sight, 62–63
        smell and taste, 59–60
        touch, 60–61
    suggestions for, 57–59
Experience of pain, 87, 88, 91, 93, 98, 100, 115

Foundation for Health, 149

Gerson Institute, 149
Gout, 100
Green, Alice and Elmer, 27, 52
Guided imagery. *See* Clinical imagery; Pain-control imagery
Guroff, Juliet J., 29

Hall, Nicholas, 52
Headaches, 89–90, 94–95, 130–33
    objective imagery and, 98, 100
Health and Human Services Department, U.S., 9–10
Hearing exercises, 61–62, 69–70
Holistic Health Havens, 149
Hypothalamus, 30–32

Imagery, 32–33, 39–86. *See also* Pain-control imagery
    of children, 56
    exercises. *See* Effective imagery exercises
    imagination compared with, 42
    involuntary response and, 46–50
    negative, 49
    relaxation and, 112–13
    sensors and, 39–40
Imagery Effectiveness Scale, 65–67, 70, 71, 94
Imaginal learning, 43–46
Immune system, 30, 52, 106
International Association for the Study of Pain (IASP), 9, 149
International Imagery Association (IIA), 150
International League Against Rheumatism 150
International Society for Imagery Science (ISIS), 145
International Society for Mental Imagery Techniques in Psychotherapy and Psychology (SITIM), 150
Interpretation of pain, 87, 88, 91–93, 100, 115
Intractable pain. *See* Pain, chronic
Involuntary functions, 36–37
Involuntary response, imagery and, 46–50

Johnson, Virginia, 49–50

Keats, John, 1

Learning, imaginal, 43–46
Liddy, G. Gordon, 26
Loeser, John, 9
Logical sequence of image, 58

McMahon, Jim, 28
Mantle, Mickey, 28
Masters, William, 49–50
Mathews-Simonton, Stephanie, 52
Medical treatment
    drugs, 11–13
    electrical stimulation, 11, 14–15
    limits of, 9, 11–16
    nerve blocks, 11, 13–14
    surgery, 11, 14
    in World War II, 26
Memory, 79–81
Migraine headaches, 89–90, 94–95,
        98, 100, 130–33
Mind, 13, 14
Mind-body connection, 25–38. *See
    also* Imagery; Pain-control
    imagery
    computer compared to, 32
    examples of, 26–29
    neurodevelopmental imperative
        theory and, 35–38
    psychosomatic pain and, 10–11
    Rossi's three-stage process of, 31
Mind modulation, 29–30
Morphine, 26, 31
Multiple personality disorder, 29

National Chronic Pain Outreach As-
    sociation (NCPO), 150
National Committee on the Treat-
    ment of Intractable Pain
    (NCTIP), 150
National Headache Foundation, 151
National Head Injury Foundation, 151
National Health Federation (NHF),
    151
National Institute of Health, 7
National Reye's Syndrome Founda-
    tion, 151

Natural Marketing Association, 151
Negative images, 49
Nerve blocks, 11, 13–14
Nervous system, 31, 34, 36–37
Neurodevelopmental imperative,
        theory of, 35–38
Nicklaus, Jack, 46
Norepinephrine, 32
Norton, Ken, 28

Objective imagery, 90, 91, 97–103,
    116
    autogenic prompt and, 98, 99–
        101
    examples of use of, 98–101
    Guide to, 99, 100
    summary of, 122–23
ODPHP National Health Informa-
        tion Center, 152
Olshan, Neil, 50
Ornstein, Robert, 37–38
Ostrander, Sheila, 44–45
Ownership of pain, 24

Pain, acute, 8
Pain, chronic (intractable pain)
    classification of, 9–11
    examples of, 17–18
    functions of, 8–9
    incidence of, 7
    perceptions of, 22–24
    psychogenic, 9–11
Pain Behavior Assessment, 19–22
Pain control, 115
    examples of, 26–29
    mind-body connection and, 25–
        38. *See also* Imagery; Mind-
        body connection; Pain-
        control imagery
    need for, 10, 11
    self-assessment and, 19–22
    taking responsibility and, 22–24
    use of, 115–24
Pain-control imagery, 50–53, 87–
    103. *See also* Imagery
    case studies of use of, 125–44
    examples of use of, 89–90, 94–
        101
    formula for, 87

Pain-control imagery (*cont.*)
  objective, 90, 91, 97–103. *See also*
      Objective imagery
  review of, 115
  subjective, 90–97, 101–2. *See also*
      Subjective imagery
Pain-Control Scale, 3–5
Pain relief, economic costs of, 7, 11
Pan American League Against Rheumatism, 152
Parasympathetic nervous system, 36
Perceptions of pain experience, 22–24
Post, Robert M., 29
Psychogenic pain, 9–11
Psychosomatic pain, 10
Putnam, Frank W., 29

Radical implantation technique, 14–15
Relaxation, 103, 105–13, 116, 121
  breathing and, 107–9
  definition of, 105
  detachment and, 109–12
  imagery and, 112–13
  what it is not, 105
Responsibility, taking, 22–24
Reynaud's syndrome, 95–96, 100, 101
Roger Wyburn-Mason and Jack M. Blount Foundation for the Eradication of Rheumatoid Disease, 152
Rossi, E. L., 29–31

Sanctuary (safe haven) technique, 119–21, 123–24, 142–44
Schroeder, Lynn, 44–45
Schwartz, Gary, 89
Schwarz, Jack, 26–27
Schwarzenegger, Arnold, 46
Self-assessment, pain control and, 19–22
Sensors, 39–40
  objective imagery and, 99
  use of, 58–59
Sensory deprivation exercises, 59–64

Sexual performance, imagery in, 50
Shealy, C. Norman, 50
Siegel, Bernie, 51
Sight, sensory deprivation exercise for, 62–63
Silberman, Edward K., 29
Simonton, Carl, 52
Smell, sensory deprivation exercise for, 59–60
Spastic colon, 100
Spatial integration, 71–74
Stoic posture, 24
Stress
  coping with. *See* Relaxation
  effects of, 106
Subjective imagery, 90–97, 101–2, 116
  autogenic prompt and, 92, 93, 95–97
  case histories of, 94–97
  Guide to, 92–93
  objective imagery compared with, 97, 98
  sanctuary (safe haven) technique, 119–21, 123–24, 142–44
  summary of, 122
Subjectivity, pain and, 25–26
Support groups and other organizations, 145–52
Surgery, 11, 14, 27–28
Sympathetic nervous system, 36

Taste, sensory deprivation exercise for, 59–60
Tesla, Nikola, 41–42
Tilney, Frederic, 38
TNS (transcutaneous nerve stimulator), 15–16
Tolerance to drugs, 13
Touch, sense of, 60–61, 68–69
Touch for Health Foundation, 152
Transcutaneous Nerve Stimulator (TNS), 15–16
Treatment, medical. *See* Medical treatment